Preparations and Uses of Chinese Medicated Spirits and Wine

Written by Lu Lei Yu Yangbo
           Lu Shuyun and Liu Hongjun
Translated by Li Yang and Jiang Xiaomei
Version Revised by Harold Swindall

Shandong Friendship Publishing House

First Edition 1996

ISBN7—80551—835—1/R · 16

Published by

Shandong Friendship Publishing House

Shengli Street, Jinan, China

Printed by

Shandong Dezhou Xinhua Printing House

Distributed by

China International Book Trading Corporation

35 Chegongzhuang Xilu, Beijing 100044, China

P. O. Box 399, Beijing, China

Printed in the People's Republic of China

Preface

Alcoholic beverages like white spirits, rice, grape or millet wine and beer are people's daily drinks.

The use of alcoholic drinks, especially spirits and wine, for the treatment of diseases was a great invention in medical history. People use medicated spirits and wine more frequently than ordinary spirits and wine to treat diseases and promote health. Medicated spirits and wine are usually made in two ways: either by infusing medicinal herbs or food in spirits or wine to obtain their useful components in the form of clear liquids, or by fermenting medicinal herbs or food directly with distiller's yeast and rice. Chinese medicated spirits and wine have a long history and are mentioned in the medical books of past dynasties. Chinese medicated spirits and wine are not simple infusions. They are made under the guidance of traditional Chinese medicinal theory to give full play to their potency in reinforcing the effect of medicinal herbs and promoting their absorption by the body. They have proved miraculously effective in treating diseases, and are a precious heritage of traditional Chinese medicine.

Chinese medicated spirits and wine are easy to make and store, and also convenient to take. With a wide variety and extensive applicability, they are people's satisfactory choices in treating diseases and promoting health. However, like any other medicines, medicated spirits and wine can do both good and harm to the human body and will produce side effects if taken inappropriately. Therefore, they should be selected and taken under a physician's direction. It is sincerely hoped that this book will give you happiness and health.

The Compilers
February 1996

Translaters' Note

Foreign readers may be confused by some of the usages found in this volume. To help clarify the terminology, "spirits" refers to Chinese white spirits made mainly from fermented sorghum. A "joss stickstick" is an incense burned in a temple. One "*cun*" equals the length of the middle phalange of the index finger. One "liang" equals the weight of 0. 05 kilogram. When the recipe specifies frying something "in a liquid," it means something other than oil, e. g, vinegar or wine. If you are unfamiliar with terms like "*qi*" and "*yang*", consult a Chinese culture reference book.

The translaters invite readers to write with questions and hope you find the book interesting reading.

Harold Swindall
Li Yang
June 1996

Contents

9

13

14

Chapter One   Invention and Application
of Alcoholic Drinks

Section One   Invention and Application of
Alcoholic Drinks

Alcoholic drinks in our country have a very long history. People in primitive society may have gotten inspirations from the natural fermentation of wild fruits and grains, but ancient documents and records are widely divided over when people started to make alcoholic drinks. Some say it was in the Xia Dynasty. For example, *Anecdotes of the Counsellors in the Warring States* says, "The princess ordered Yidi to make wine to present to Yu." Others maintain it was in the Shang Dynasty and still others hold it was in the Zhou Dynasty, asserting, "Dukang invented spirit." The earthenware wine vessels unearthed in the ruins of the Longshang Culture show that alcoholic drinks came into being no later than the Xia Dynasty. Jiangtong in the Jin Dynasty said in his *Admonition on Alcoholic Drinks*, "The invention of alcoholic drinks is attributed to the Creator ··· leftovers from meals which had been disposed of in the open and had accumulated for a long period of time sent forth fragrance and turned into wine, thus the origin of alcoholic drinks." That shows that boiled cereals disposed of in the open can ferment into wine under certain natural conditions. The agricultural production of the Shang Dynasty developed remarkably and the oracle bone inscriptions in the dynasty record many varieties of crops including standing grain, wheat, broomcorn millet, millet and rice. The increase of crops laid down a material foundation for the prosperity of the wine-making industry. Alcoholic drinks were popular in the Shang Dynasty. The bronze vessels unearthed in the ruins of the Shang Dynasty include many wine vessels and that points to a large-scale wine-making industry at that time. The Shang people offered wines as sacrifices and used wines to treat diseases.

The application of alcoholic drinks to medical treatment is a great invention in medical history. They were the earliest stimulants (used in small quantities) and anesthetics (used in large quantities), could promote blood circulation, function as medicines and be used as solutions. It bacame a common occurrence that later generations used wines to prepare herbal medicine. As people's medical knowledge and experience in using medicines, and the varieties of medicines were enriched, their ability to treat diseases with wine and spirit and medicated wine and spirit developed. *The Yellow Emperor's Canon of Internal Medicine* mentions the fact that ancient people "made medicated wine," points out its therapeutic effect and says, "Pathogens attack people frequently and it is perfect prevention to take wines." *A History of the Han Dynasties* holds that alcoholic drinks top all other medicines.

Dosage form refers to the form of medical preparations. Because traditional Chinese medicines are numerous, have different properties and very complex reactions to one another, and are used compositely and under varied clinical demands, they must be prepared in certain dosage forms in order to raise their potency, reduce their toxity and make them safe, effective and convenient to take.

In addition to their medical value, alcoholic drinks are very good mixing solutions, so they and medicated spirits and wine became important components of the dosage forms of traditional Chinese medicines. Medicated spirits and wine are made by infusing pieces of traditional Chinese medicines in spirits or yellow rice or millet wine to obtain their active components in the form of clear liquids either for oral administration or for external use. The spirit of Chinese fevervine in *The Yellow Emperor's Canon* and the spirit of *Erigeron elongatus Ledeb.* in *Synopsis of Prescriptions of the Golden Chamber* are the earliest medicated spirits to have been recorded in ancient medical books. In addition to medicated spirits and wine, there are also tinctures, spirits and elixirs that can be used to treat diseases. A tincture is made by infusing traditional Chinese medicines in alcohol of a certain proof to obtain their active components in the form of liquid. Spirit is an alcohol solution with a certain proof containing fragrant and volatile medicines. An elixir is a medicated alcohol solution containing sugar. They are all similar to medicated spirits and wine.

Section Two　Introduction to Alcoholic Drinks

1. Alcoholic Drinks

Alcoholic drinks are made from fermented sorghum, barley, rice, millet, grapes and other fruits into spirits, yellow rice or millet wine, beer and grape wine, etc.

They have always been able to do both harm and good to health and modern medicine has proved that.

Ancient chinese people held that spirit and wine "bitter, sweet, pungent, toxic and very hot in nature, can function as medicine to eliminate all pathogenic factors, dredge the channels, nourish the spleen, the stomach and the skin and dispel depression, but intemperance is prone to shorten one's life, impair his vitality and distort his nature " (*Essentials of Diet*, vol. 3, Spirit). Tao Hongjing in the Liang Dynasty concluded that the reason why "great cold freezes all liquids including the sea except spirit and wine" is that spirit and wine are hot and that pharmacists and physicians made up medicated spirit and wine or prescribed medicated spirit and wine simply because they wanted to make use of their heat to treat diseases and to "give play to their medical potency." He also pointed out, "Intemperance does harm to health because spirit and wine are toxic." In *Compendium of Materia Medica*, Li Shizhen said, "Spirit and wine are heavenly drinks. If taken in moderation, they will promote the flow of *qi* and blood, dispel cold and depression and be refreshing, but they will impair vital essence and the stomach, consume blood unduly and induce phlegm-fire if taken intemperately"; furthermore, "Spirit and wine are very hot in nature, so they are toxic."

Essentials of Promoting Health says, "Spirits and wine do both good and harm to health. … long-standing intemperance weakens *qi* and vigour, so caution should be taken." Although ancient Chinese people did not know that spirits and wine partially consist of alcohol, they drew the conclusion after observing the influence of spirits and wine in all their manifestations that spirits and wine have warming property and are toxic, can dredge the channels, nourish the spleen and the stomach, dispel depression and function as medicine. Thus, temperate drinking does good to health, and medicated spirits and wine can be used to treat diseases. They also pointed out that because spirits and wine have warming property and are toxic, intemperance shortens one's life, weakens his vigour and distorts his nature, so they warned people against addiction.

Modern medical research finds that spirits and wine partially consist of alcohol. They have a wide variety and their composition is strikingly different. Distilled alcoholic drinks like sorghum spirit have higher amounts of alcohol, fatty acids, fats and aldehydes and their alcohol content is higher than that of those not distilled, e.g. yellow rice or millet wine and grape wine, which have glucose, dextrin and glycerin in addition to water and alcohol.

Alcoholic drinks have no nutrients except beer and grape wine and other fruit wine. Alcohol produces heat for only a short time and after that a lot of glucose in the human body is consumed. According to a test, 500 grams of white spirit wastes one half to two thirds of a person's daily intake of heat. The burning of one kilogram of alcohol in the body produces 7. 1 Kilocalories of heat.

In the body, alcohol has an influence on the central nervous system. similar to that of an anaesthetic. It also weakens behavioral inhibitions and causes excitement. A moderate quantity of alcohol can dilate blood vessels, thus reddening the skin and giving one a sensation of warmth, while an undue quantity of it paralyses the medullary center, thus inducing collapse.

Alcoholic drinks with a low content of alcohol can promote the secretion of gastric fluid and acid and the digestion while those with a high alcohol content irritate the gastric mucosa strongly and damage the mouth cavity, the stomach and the intestinal mucosa. Frequent irritations of the gastric and intestinal mucosa from long-standing alcohol addiction cause chronic inflammation and affect digestion, thus bringing about denutrition, pancreatitis, esophagus inflammation and gastric and duodenal ulcers.

The metabolism of the heat produced by alcohol in the liver can induce pathologic changes there such as alcoholic hepatitis, fatty liver and cirrhosis.

Topical application of alcohol to the skin can speed up the volitilization of internal heat and can be used to lower the temperature of a patient running a high fever. High proof alcohol can dehydrate cellular plasmogen and cause precipitation, thus performing apocrustic and stimulating functions. Medical alcohol with a concentration of 75% can be used as disinfectant.

Alcoholic drinks can also affect the lungs. Zhu Zhenxiang

said that spirits and wine "are volatile, so *qi* easily volatilizes with them. As a result, phlegm stagnates in the upper part of the body while urine retention occurs in the lower part, pathogenic wind and cold invade, heat stagnates in the interior and the lung-*qi* is impaired. " Spirits and wine irritate the respiratory tract and weaken its defensive function.

Alcohol addiction does harm to heart patients in particular. Alcoholic drinks, especially hard liquor, can speed up the heart rate, dilate the heart and weaken the contracting function of the cardiac muscle. The chronic alcoholic also has blurred vision, mental deficiency and dizziness, etc. Intoxication does serious harm to the human body and can even paralyze the respiratory and circulatory functions.

If pregnant women drink too much, especially when they are at the initial stage of pregnancy, they risk giving birth to babies with very small heads, eyes and legs, defective hearts and mental retardation.

People have paid attention to the influence of alcoholic drinks on sex since ancient times. In *Macbeth*, a guard remarks that much drink "provokes the desire, but it takes away the performance. " Modern medicine has proved the playwright's observation. Even if the alcoholic proof of a certain drink is not high enough to make people drunk, it can dramatically check the erection of the penis or negatively effect the pulsation of the vagina. The cause of this effect may be that alcohol as a check on the central nervous system disturbs the transmission of the reaction induced by sexual excitement. In addition, in recent years it has been discovered that alcohol can lower the level of testosterone and progesterone even of a young and healthy man. Some data show that 50% of male and 25% of female alcoholics have a sexual dysfunction.

However, the acute effect of alcohol on sex is more complicated than the fact mentioned above. Some people think that alcohol has a "non-inhibitory" effect. In other words, alcohol can reduce the sexual inhibition an individual usually has, so it can relax some people and strengthen their sexual desire. Therefore, the effect of alcohol on the sexual function of individuals varies greatly and has much to do with the quantity of spirits, wine and beer taken, occasions and moods. However, one thing is clear: if one gets too drunk, he will not be able to have any sex at all.

People have been concerned about whether hypertension patients can drink. A folk remedy prescribing 10 grams of cleaned and minced chrysanthemun flowers decoted in a certain amount of glutinous rice wine and taken twice a day is used to treat the liver heat type hypertension and dizziness. Recent clinical researches have discoved that drinking moderately can increase the high-density lipoprotein in the blood, prevent low density lipoproteins and cholesterol from depositing on the vascular walls and is conducive to preventing atherosclerosis. Spirits have a high alcohol content and can do harm to health and speed up atheroclerosis if taken for a long period of time.

To sum up, alcoholic drinks do both good and harm to health, depending not only on how much and how long one drinks, but also on the occasion and mood. Supposing the suitable intake of spirit, wine or beer of a normal person is 1 gram per 1,000 grams of body weight, he can drink 100 grams of spirit, or

300 grams of grape wine or 2 liters of beer a day. However, the intake should depend on an individual's constitution and the general principle is that one had better drink in moderation.

2. Grape Wine

Grape wine is a drink with a low alcohol content. According to *Essentials of Diet*, grape wine "replenishes *qi*, regulates the middle-*jiao*, strengthens one's endurance for hunger and fortifies one's will. " Recent research shows that grape wine contains 32 kinds of amino acids, 12 kinds of vitamins and a few kinds of nitrogenous nutrients. Because it is rich in Vitamin B12 and benzonic acid, a moderate intake of it can replenish blood and increase its high density lipoproteins so that the incidence of coronary disease and cerebrovascular disease is reduced. Grape wine is sweet in taste, warm in property, beautiful in color and easily intoxicates people but its effect is easy to dispel. It is also tonic and nutritious.

3. Beer

Beer is made from the fermented mix of saccharified barley and supplementary ingredients, hops and yeast and contains 10— 12% alcohol, saccharides, 17 kinds of amino acids and 10 kinds of vitamins essential to the human body. Rich in vitamin B, it is called "fluid bread. " 1 litre of beer produces 760 Kilocalories of heat equal to those produced by 5 or 6 eggs. Most of the starch in the raw materials of beer is transformed into glucose and maltose that can be directly absorbed by the human body and a small part of it is changed into alcohol and carbon dioxide, which perform the functions of exciting the nerves, replenishing *qi*, regulating blood circulation and promoting digestion.

The agreeable bitter taste of beer comes from its hops, which mainly consist of aromatic resin, bitter flavoring, tannin, proteins and glucose etc, which are the major raw materials of beer. The components of hops not only give beer a unique taste, but also perform the functions of reducing fever, relieving urine retention, tonifying the heart and tranquilizing the mind.

Practice has proved drinking beer frequently and moderately not only provides the body with abundant nutrients, but also regulates physiological function and metabolism and has certain medical effect on hypertension, arteriosclerorsis, cardiac diseases, hydrorenal disease and tuberculosis.

4. Medicated Spirits and Wine

In medicine, besides using spirits, yellow rice or millet wine, grape wine and beer directly to treat diseasse, we use medicated spirits and wine more frequently. They can do both good and harm to the human body, but we can make good use of them by infusing medicinal herbs in them to extract the herbs' medical essence, give play to their potency with the help of the spirit and wine and promote its absorption by the human body so that its miraculous effects in treating diseases are shown.

Medicated spirit and wine differ in variety and property and the patient can choose the one suitable to his disease.

Chapter Two Preparation of Medicated Spirits and Wine and Principles of Their Application

Section One Preparation of Medicated Spirits and Wine

1. Selection of Spirits and Wine

The selection of spirits and wine depends on their properties and a patient's illness. Spirits and wine are made in different ways.

Wine is made from various kinds of brewed, fermented and filtrated starchy and saccharine materials, e. g. yellow rice or millet and grape wine. The alcohol content is usually low, below 20%.

Spirits are made from fermented and distilled starchy and saccharine materials not filtrated, e. g. hard liquor. The alcohol content is usually high, from 38% to 55%.

Spirits and wine can be judged and chosen according to their color, smell and taste. The color of good spirit and wine should be normal. For example, the spirit in our country is usually colorless although sometimes it is light yellow. Fruit wine should have the color of the fruit it is made from. Good spirit should be "lustrous like silver light" and have a heavy fragrance that is refreshing while a bad one has an irritating smell. Good spirit and wine taste "as sweet as milk," and "as pungent as ginger, as sweet as honey and as bitter as gall." That is to say, they should have the five flavours of sweetness, sourness, bitterness, pungence and fragrance.

2. Getting Medicines Ready

Get ready the medicines prescribed either by a physician or in a medical book. After that, remove the impurities. Some of them need processing (such as washing, cleaning, discarding the useless parts, cutting into small pieces, soaking in water, drying in the sun, steaming, stir-baking) first and this can be done according to local processing methods and experience.

3. Preparation of Medicated Spirits and Wine

(1) Decoction

Crush the prescribed medicinal ingredients together into lumps, put them into a pot, add water (it should submerge the ingredients by 6-10 cm.), infuse the ingredients for 4—6 hours, decoct them for 1-2 hours, filtrate them, decoct them again, filtrate them, mix the filtrates, and let the mixture sit for 6-10 hours. Remove the settled dregs, boil down the clear liquid (5 kg. of raw materials are usually boiled down to 1.5-2.5 kg. of clear and thick liquid). Add spirits containing 50%-60% alcohol in equal quantity when the clear liquid cools down. Mix them well, put the mixture into a bottle or a mug, keep it sealed hermetically for about 7 days, then remove the dregs, filtrate the clear liquid and seal up the bottle.

With only a small quantity of spirits, thereis not a strong taste of spirits. However, volatile fragrant medicinal ingredients are not fit for decoction in this way.

(2) Extraction by Infusion

a. Extraction by Cold Infusion

Crush the prescribed medicinal ingredients, put them into a cloth bag, put the bag into a container, add spirit or yellow rice or millet wine of the prescribed quantity (usually 4—6 times the ingredients), then seal up the container. The duration of the infusion depends on the properties of the ingredients and the requirements of the prescription, usually for about half a month, or longer in winter. Extract the ingredients, filtrate the extract, settle the filtrate, put it into a bottle and seal it up.

b. Extraction by Hot Infusion

Crush the prescribed ingredients, put them into a container, add spirits containing about 50% alcohol (usually 4—6 times the ingredients or according to the prescription), and put the container into a larger container with water. Heat the ingredients for a short time (otherwise the spirits will volatize) till they bubble, remove the container from the fire, and pour the ingredients and the spirits into a container with a big mouth, sealing it up while they are still hot. Keep them for 10—15 days, then draw the clear liquid, press the dregs, mix their extract with the clear liquid and pour the mixture into a bottle.

Extraction by hot infusion needs no complicated equipment. This method is simple and suitable for medicinal ingredients in particular that have a lot of starch and resin.

(3) Brewing

Decoct the prescribed ingredients in water, filtrate tnem, remove the dregs and boil down the filtrate. Some medicinal ingredients like mulberry fruit, pears and bayberry fruit can be pressed to obtain their extract directly. Mix the extract with steamed glutinous rice and spirits, pour the mixture into a clean container, seal it up and keep it airtight for 4—6 days at an appropriate temperature.

(4) Percolation

Percolation refers to the method of using a solution to extract active principles from medicinal ingredients or food through a percolator. This method is efficient since it saves solution, so it is frequently used. However, do not use a highly volatile solution. The solutions frequently used are alcohols of different proofs, acid water or alkaline water, etc.

a. The equipment for percolation usually consists of a percolator and a receiving flask. The percolator is made either of metal, enamel or glass, is either a cylinder or a cone in shape and the opening at its bottom is linked with a rubber tube with a spiral clip which is used to control the speed of flow of the percolation.

The selection of a percolator depends on the expansion of the crushed medicinal ingredients. Highly expandible ingredients are not suitable for the alcohol of high proof.

b. sift the prescribed and crushed ingredients through a sieve of 30 meshes, put them into a container, add solution of equal quantity, mix them well and hermetically seal the container to let the ingredients infuse and expand to the full. The duration depends on the properties of the ingredients, usually 1—4 hours.

Now wrap a lump of absorbent cotton in absorbent gauze, wet it with solution and put it under the opening at the bottom of the percolator. Put the infused ingredients into the percolator, spreading each layer evenly and flattening them with a flat utensil. If the solution's alcohol content is high, press them compactly; press them loosely if the water content is high. When all the ingredients have been put into the percolator layer upon layer, cover them with 2—3 layers of gauze, lay clean glass balls or other weights that do not react upon the solution, connect the receiving flask with the opening and loosen the spiral clip on the rubber tube. Then add the solution slowly, tighening the clip when solution flows from the opening. Pour the solution back into the percolator, add more solution till the solution in the percolator submerges the ingredients and is 5—10 cm. above then. Cover the percolator and let it sit for 24—28 hours or for a prescribed period of time.

Loosen the spiral clip to start percolation. Unless prescribed otherwise, the flow rate of percolation per kilogram is 1—3 ml, or 3—5 ml. During percolation, keep adding solution to keep the solution level in the percolator at a certain height and stop the percolation when colorless and odorless percolate flows out. Press the dregs to obtain their extract, mix the extract and the percolate, then keep the mixture static for 24 hours to settle it. Finally, filtrate it.

Of the four methods mentioned above, extraction by infusion is the most frequently used while percolation is only applied to industrial mass production.

4. Administration

Medicated spirits and wine had better be taken while they are warm so as to give play to their potency. Tonic medicated spirits and wine can be taken slowly at dinner. Medical experts hold that a healthy person's proper daily intake of medicated spirit or wine is generally 1 gram per kilogram of body weight. However, an individual's daily intake of medicated spirits and wine should depend on his constitution and the properties of the medicated spirits or wine he is to take.

Medicated spirits and wine can also be applied topically to an affected part of the body several times a day.

5. Storage

Because medicated spirits and wine contain alcohol, they do not go bad easily; even so, they should be stored in an airtight container at a low temperature and protected from light to prevent the alcohol in them from volatilizing, settling and going bad. If there is a lot of precipitation in medicated spirits and wine, they should not be taken until they pass medical inspection and are filtrated again.

6. Cautions

The intake of medicated spirits and wine should be moderate and the patient who has a fever, night sweats of flushing zygomatic region due to extreme internal heat caused by *yin* deficiency, or who is thin and weak should be cautious in taking medicated spirits and wine because they are pungent, warm and dry and transmit heat easily and impair body fluids. The patient suffering from hepatitis, cirrhosis, peptic ulcer, infiltrative or cavitary tuberculosis, epilepsy, cardiac insufficiency, chronic nephritis or chronic colitis should not take them, let alone those allergic to them. Pregnant women must not take them. See Chapter One: Alcoholic Drinks.

Section Two   Principles of the Application of Medicated Spirits and Wine

The application of medicated spirits and wine to the treatment of diseases is similar to that of Chinese drugs. Medicated spirits and wine differ in variety, composition, properties and use; therefore, their application should be based on the theory of Chinese medicine. Only when they are based on certain principles and used properly can they cure patients of diseases; otherwise, they will do harm instead of good. They should be used flexibly and appropriately according to the following principles:

1. Medicated spirits and wine should be chosen in the light of the conditions of the body and be congenial to *qi*. A healthy person, whose *yin* and *yang* are in equilibrium, whose blood and *qi* are in order and who leads a normal life can take healthy medicated spirits or wine. A person who has no clinical symptoms, but whose *yin* and *yang* are imbalanced and who has either cold or heat in the interior should take the medicated spirits or wine for cold or heat. *Yin* and *yang* can be balanced by treating cold syndrome with warming drugs and treating heat syndrome by using cooling drugs.

2. Medicated spirits and wine should be chosen in the light of the nature and symptoms of a disease. In treatment, pathological conditions should be analyzed and differentiated according to the classification of eight principal syndromes, namely the syndromes of *yin* and *yang*; interior and exterior; cold and heat; or deficiency and excess. At the same time, attention should be paid to the treatment of a disease with recipes and drugs opposite to its symptoms, the treatment of both the primary and the secondary aspects of a disease and the reinforcement and purging of the viscera.

(1) A disease can be treated with recipes and drugs opposite to its symptoms. For example, cold syndrome can be treated with warming drugs and deficiency syndrome can be treated with reinforcing drugs. A disease can also be treated contrary to the routine. In some special cases, illness of the deficiency type can be treated by purgation; excess syndrome with tonifying method; cold syndrome can be treated with cooling drugs and heat syndrome with warming drugs. The therapy is used in the light of recognizing the signs and symptoms correctly; knowing clearly whether they are deceptive or not (a disease of the cold type may have heat symptoms and a disease of heat type may have cold symptoms); and making full use of the properties of medicated spirits and wine (warming spirits and wine can go with cooling drugs) to suit them to different diseases.

(2) A physician should differentiate the symptoms and causes of a disease, know clearly whether it is acute or chronic and treat it under the guidance of the principle of "giving priority to the treatment of the symptoms of an acute disease and the causes

of a chronic one. "For example, one can take mild tonic medicated spirits or wine to reinforce the fundamentas to prolong life.

3. Medicated spirits and wine should be used flexibly in the light of time, place and a patient's conditions. Patients of different sexes and ages should take different medicated spirits and wine in different seasons and places and adjust their administrations and dosage accordingly.

4. One should take medicated spirits or wine in moderation. Medicated spirit and wine can treat diseases, promote health and prolong life, but they can also do harm because of the properties of their ingredients. One should take medicated spirit or wine in moderation, follow the physician's directions strictly and not exceed the right dosage.

5. Priority should be given to disease prevention. Medicated spirits and wine are mostly tonic and can meet people's demand for longevity, but it should be pointed out that the nourishment of the human body should vary with the change of *yin* and *yang* in the four seasons.

Chapter Three   Application of Medicated Spirits and Wine

Section One   Lung Carbuncle

The clinical symptoms of carbuncle are a cough, chest pain, fever and expectoration of phlegm and even pus and blood. These are similar to the symptoms of pulmonary abscess, suppurative pneumonia, bronchiecchus and bronchial infection and suppuration in modern medicine. Carbuncle usually has the stages of exterior syndrome, pyogenesis and ulceration.

1. Spirit of *Senecio Integrifolius*

Ingredients:

Senecio integrifolius 15 grams, Chinese osbeckia 15 grams.

Pharmaceutical Process:

Put the herbs and 250 grams of spirits into a pot, put the pot into a larger container with water and decoct the ingredients.

Indication:

Pulmonary suppuration.

Administration and Dosage:

1 dose per day till recovery.

Source:

Jiaochuan Commune of Zhuchang County, Zhejiang Province, *Selection of the Materials of the National Exhibition of*

Chinese Medicinal Herbs and New Therapy, 1972, P. 138.

2. Wine of *Verbena Officinalis*

Ingredients:

Verbena officinalis 90 grams, rhizome of tiangengyazhi 60 grams, Cordate houttuynia 60 grams, *Aristolochia mollicissima Hance* 45 grams, cogongrass rhizome 45 grams.

Pharmaceutical Process:

Wash the herbs clean and dry them in sunlight. Decoct them in 1,000 grams of sweet wine with 500 grams of water in which rice has been washed and 50—200 grams of wine over a slow fire and boil down the decoction to 1,100ml.

Indication:

Pulmonary suppuration.

Administration and Dosage:

Take 100ml of it the first time and 80ml thereafter before breakfast and supper.

Caution:

Do not eat sour and pungent food while taking the wine.

Source:

Xiangyang County and Yicheng County, Hubei Province, *Selection of the Materials of the National Exhibition of Chinese Medicinal Herbs and New Therapy*, 1972, P. 137

3. Wine of *Tiejiaojiangjun*

Ingredients:

Tiejiaojiangjun

Pharmaceutical Process:

Wash the rhizome clean and dry it in sunlight. Cut off the rootlets, mince it and put 250 grams of it into an earthenware pot. Add 1,250 grams of yellow millet wine or water, seal up the pot with bamboo leaves, put the pot into a larger container with water and decoct the ingredients over a slow fire for 3 hours. When there is about 1,000ml. of extract in the pot, add antiseptic to it.

Indication:

Pulmonary suppuration.

Administration and Dosage:

20—40ml doses according to the patient's age and condition, 3 times per day. It is usually taken with water, but if the patient runs a continuous high fever, has difficulty expectorating stenchy phlegm and the disease is lingering, it should be taken with wine.

Source:

Hospital of Nantong City, Jiangsu Province, *Selection of the Materials of the National Exhibition of Chinese Medicinal Herbs and New Therapy*, 1972, p. 137.

Section Two Cough and Asthmoid Respiration

Cough and asthmoid respiration are the major symptoms of a lung disease. Cough includes tussiculation and coughing phlegm from the lungs. Asthmoid respiration is characterized by short breath and laryngeal whistling rale. Cough and asthmoid respiration are similar to acute or chronic bronchitis and bronchial asthma in modern medicine.

1. Spirit of Black Nightshade Fruit

Ingredients:

Black nightshade fruit 250 grams.

Pharmaceutical Process:

Let the ripe fruit infuse in 500 grams of spirits for 20—30 days.

Actions:

Dispels heat, removes pathogenic factors, promotes diuresis and subdues swelling.

Indication:

Chronic bronchitis.

Administration and Dosage:

Oral administration, 1 spoon each time 3 times per day.

Source:

Materia Medica of Jilin, 1971, p. 39

2. Spirit of Rhamus

Ingredients:

Rhamus seed 60 grams.

Pharmaceutical Process:

Let the seed infuse in 500 grams of spirit for 5 days.

Actions:

Relieves cough and reduces sputum.

Indications:

Chronic bronchitis and pneumonectasis.

Administration and Dosage:

Oral administration, 1 teaspoon 3 times per day.

Source:

Research Institute of Chinese Medicine and Medicinal Herbs of Jilin Province, *Shandong Medicine*, No. 1, 1971, p. 2

3. Drink of *Rhododendron Micranthum Turcz*

Ingredients:

Fresh leaves of *Rhododendrom micranthum Turcz* 1,350

grams.

Pharmaceutical Process:

Let the leaves infuse in 15 litres of spirits containing 50% alcohol and 10 litres of water for 5 days and then make a 30% concentration drink with them.

Actions:

Relieves cough and reduces sputum.

Indications:

Senile chronic bronchitis.

Administration and Dosage:

5—15ml dose, 3 times per day 30 minutes after each meal. 7—10 days constitute a course of treatment.

Cautions:

Do not take other medicine for bronchitis while taking the spirits.

Source:

Clinical Observation and Experimental Research of the Treatment of Chronic Bronchitis with Rhododendron Micranthum Turcz, ed. Cooperation Group of Research of the Treatment and Prevention of Chronic Bronchitis of Dalian Branch of Shenyang Railway Bureau, 1972, p. 1.

4. Cough and Asthma Spirit

Ingredients:

Piper *kadssura Ohwi* 60 grams,

Pharmaceutical Process:

Let them soak in cold spirits.

Indications:

bronchitis and bronchial asthma.

Administration and Dosage:

10ml dose before breakfast and supper. Do not heat it, otherwise it will lose its effectiveness.

Source:

Hongwei Pharmaceutical Factory of Taigu, Shanxi Province, *Selection of the Materials of the National Exhibition of Chinese Medicinal Herbs and New Therapy*, 1972, p. 138.

5. Spirit of *Crotataria Ferruginea Grah*

Ingredients:

Crotataria ferruginea Grah. (dried) 120 grams.

Pharmaceutical Process:

Let it soak in 1,000 grams of spirits for 7 days.

Indication:

Tuberculosis.

Administration and Dosage:

8ml per dose, three times per day.

Source:

The People's Hospital of Sangzhi County, Hunan Province, *Selection of the Materials of the National Exhibition of Chinese Medicinal Herbs and New Therapy*, 1972, p. 138.

6. Wine of Stemona Root

Ingredients:

Stemona root.

Pharmaceutical Process:

Cut the root into slices and parch them. Then put them into a bag and let them soak in wine.

Indications:

Chronic or acute cough.

Administration and Dosage:

A small quantity each time and taken frequently.

Source:

A Handbook of Family Dietetic Therapy, 1982, p. 515.

7. Wine of Purple Perilla Seeds

Ingredients:

Purple perilla seeds 600 grams, yellow rice or millet wine 2,500 grams.

Pharmaceutical Process:

Parch the seeds for a short while, put them into a bag and let them soak in the wine for 7 days.

Indications:

Phlegm and saliva stagnancy and asthma caused by adverse rising of the lung-*qi*.

Administration and Dosage:

10ml dose, twice per day.

Source:

Encyclopedia of Chinese Diet Therapy, 1988, p. 657.

8. Wine of Citron

Ingredients:

Citron quantum satis.

Pharmaceutical Process:

Let it soak in wine.

Actions:

Strengthens the stomach and replenishes *qi*.

Administration and Dosage:

Take it frequently.

Source:

9. Wine of Mulberry Bark

Ingredients:

Mulberry bark 200 grams, millet wine 1,000 grams.

Pharmaceutical Process:

Let the minced bark soak in the wine for 7 days.

Indications:

Cough and asthma due to heat in the lungs.

Administration and Dosage:

20ml doses, 3 times per day.

Source:

Criteria of Treatment

10. Wine of Sheep Pancreas

Ingredients:

One sheep pancreas, forty Ziziphus jujube (minced) fruits, 10kgs of millet wine.

Pharmaceutical Process:

Let the pancreas and fruits soak in the wine for 7 days.

Indications:

Lingering cough due to chronic bronchitis.

Administration and Dosage:

30ml doses, 3 times per day.

Source:

A Handbook of Prescriptions for Emergencies

11. Spirits of Chinese Yam

Ingredients:

Chinese yam 15 grams, dogwood fruit 15 grams, schisandra fruit 15 grams, lucid ganoderma 15 grams, spirits 1,000 grams

Pharmaceutical Process:

Let the herbs soak in the spirits for 1 month.

Indications:

deficiency of *yin* of the lungs and the kidneys, cough due to consumption, xerostomia due to lack of body fluid, night sweating and spermatorrhea.

Administration and Dosage:

10ml doses, twice per day.

Source:

Tonic Medicine and Food

12. Wine of Geckoes

Ingredients:

2 geckoes.

Pharmaceutical Process:

Remove their heads, legs and spots, cut them into small pieces and let them soak in 500 grams of millet wine for 7 days.

Actions:

Tonifies the lungs and kidneys, improves inspiration by invigorating the kidney-*qi*, and relieves asthma.

Indications:

Consumptive disease, cough, lack of *qi* and impotence.

Administration and Dosage:

30 gram doses, twice per day.

Source:

Tonic Medicine and Food

13. Wine of Scallion and Soybeans

Ingredients:

Raw scallion 30 grams, prepared soybeans 15 grams, millet

wine 50 grams.

Pharmaceutical Process:

put the soybeans into an aluminum pot, add a small bowl of water and decoct them for 10 minutes. Add the washed scallion, decoct for five minutes, then add the wine and pour the decoction into a bowl immediately. Drink it while it is still hot.

Actions:

Induces diaphoresis, dispels exopathogens and cold and regulates the stomach.

Indications:

Wind-cold due to exopathy, fever, headache, nausea, vomiting and cough.

Administration and Dosage:

Take it while it is still hot.

Source:

Prescriptions of Meng Shen

14. Tonic Spirit

Ingredients:

Chinese angelica 960 grams; 120 grams each of the following: rhizome of ligusticum, dried orange peel, safflower, rhizome of nutgrass flatsedge, rhizome of cyathula, magnolia bark, rhizome of polygonatum and rhizome of slender acanthopanax; 240 grams each: root of herbaceous peony, prepared rhizome of rehmannia, rhizome of large-headed atractylodes, peach kernels, root of purple-flowered peucedanum, fruit of evodia, rhizome of *Alpinia officinarum Hance*, aniseed, bark of eucommia, teasel root, large-leaved gentian, rhizome of heracleum, seeds of Chinese dodder, tiger bone, fruit of Chinese wolfberry, stem of desertliving cistanche, root of narrow-leaved polygala, cores of Ziziphus jujubc, rhizome of asparagus, tuber of dwarf lilyturf, apricot kernels, schisandra fruit, wrinkled giant hyssop, Tiantai lindera root, root of Dahurian angelica, frankincense, myrrh, dried bark of *Cinnamomum cassia*, licorice root, amomum fruit and fruit of flowering quince; root of *Codonopsis pilosula* and Chinese ephedra; 180 grams each; cloves, dried fruit of zikou, sandalwood, root of *Asarum heteropides mandshuricum*, aucklandia root and Chinese prickly ash seed; 60 grams each; spirits 5,200 grams, honey 4,000 grams.

Indications:

Cough, dyspnea, abundant expectoration, short breath, chest and hypochondrium congestion, discomfort in the gastric cavity and abdomen, cold-sensitive lingering soreness in the waist and pain in the legs, menoxenia and sensation of cold and abdomen congestion.

Administration and Dosage:

Oral administration, 15 warm doses in the morning and evening.

Source:

Dispensary of Chinese Herbal and Prepared Medicine, 1991, p. 489

Cautions:

Pregnant women must not take it; healthy people should also be cautious and not eat raw or cold food while taking it.

15. Cold and Cough Spirit

Ingredients:

Lithospermum erythrorrhision 120 grams; apricot kernels,

Trichosanthes kirilowi, *Fritillaria thunbergii*, tuber of pinellia 30 grams each; dried orange peel 60 grams; *Poria cocos* and dried ginger 30 grams each; root of *Asarum heterothropolides mandshuricum* and schisandra fruit 15 grams each; root of stemona, rhizome of *Cynanchum glaucescens* and root of balloonflower 30 grams each; seeds of round cardamom 15 grams; fruit of *Poncirus trifoliata* 30 grams; longuat leaves and mulberry bark 30 grams each; fencao 15 grams; spirit 5,000 grams.

Pharmaceutical Process:

Let the herbs soak in the spirit for 10 days.

Actions:

Dispels cold and relieves cough and phlegm.

Indications:

Cold, cough, expectoration of abundant, clear and thin phlegm, dyspnea, chest congestion, fever, aversion to cold, anhidrosis, moist and smooth fur on the tongue and a tense, forceful and floating pulse felt at *cun* and *chi* locations.

Administration and Dosage:

Oral administration, 30—60ml doses, twice per day.

Source:

Dispensary of Chinese Herbal and Prepared Medicine, 1991, p. 409.

Section Three   Mumps

The clinical symptoms of mumps are fever and painful swelling in the neck; children 5—9 years old are susceptible to the disease. In modern medicine, mumps are known as epidemic parotitis caused by the mumps virus.

1. Spirit of Birthwood

Ingredients:

Rhizome of birthwood and rhizome of mountain creeper (peeled) *qs*.

Pharmaceutical Process:

Grind them with 18 grams of spirits.

Indication:

Epidemic parotitis.

Administration and Dosage:

Oral administration, one 6 gram dose per day and then continuous application of it to the affected part for 1 hour.

Source:

The Station of Public Health of Chenzhou Town, Hunan Province, *Selection of the Materials of the National Exhibition of Chinese Medicinal Herbs and New Therapy*, 1972, p. 21.

Section Four　Epigastralgia

The major symptom of epigastralgia are frequent pains near the scrobiculus cordis in the upper part of the abdomen. It often occurs in acute or chronic gastritis, gastric and dodenal ulcer, gastric neurosis and gastric cancer, etc.

1. Spirit of Hickory Nuts

Ingredients:

Hickory nuts 6,000 grams.

Pharmaceutical Process:

Pound the nuts to pieces, let them soak in 10,000 grams of spirits for 20 days till the spirits turn dark brown, filtrate the medicated spirit to remove the dregs and pour it into a bottle.

Actions:

Astriction, anti-inflammation and alleviation.

Indication:

Chronic and acute gastritis.

Administration and Dosage:

Oral administration, 10—15 ml. per dose.

Source:

Office of the Exhibition of Chinese Medicinal Herbs and New Therapy of Heilongjiang Province, *Selection of the Materials of the Exhibition of Chinese Medicinal Herbs and New Therapy*, 1970.

2. Spirit of Birthwort

Ingredients:

Rhizome of birthwort 30—60 grams.

Pharmaceutical Process:

Let the washed slices of the rhizome soak in 250 grams of spirits.

Indication:

Acute gastritis.

Administration and Dosage:

5ml doses, 2—3 times per day.

Source:

Enshi Prefecture, Hubei Province, *Selection of the Materials of the National Exhibition of Chinese Medicinal Herbs and New Therapy*, 1972, p. 154.

3. Spirit for Stomachache

Ingredients:

Garden burnet 64 grams, birthwood 64 grams, spirits 1,000

ml.

Pharmaceutical Process:

Mince the herbs and infuse them in the spirits.

Actions:

Promotes the circulation of qi, subdues swelling and alleviates pain.

Indication:

Chronic gastritis.

Administration and Dosage:

Oral administration, 10ml doses in the morning and in the evening.

Source:

Rural Preparations of Chinese Herbal Medicine of Guizhou, 1977, p. 201.

4. Spirit of Walnuts

Ingredients:

Walnuts (green) 250 grams, rhizome of *Rosa roxburghii Tratt* 130 grams, spirits 1,000 grams.

Pharmaceutical Process:

Mince the herbs and let them infuse in the cold spirits for 20 days.

Actions:

Replenishes qi, allays inflammation and alleviates pain.

Indications:

Chronic enterogastritis and abdominal pains.

Administration and Dosage:

Oral administration, 10ml doses, 3 times per day.

Remarks:

The green nuts should be pounded to pieces when used.

Source:

Rural Preparations of Chinese Herbal Medicine of Guizhou, 1977, p. 201.

5. Spirit of Fingered Citron

Ingredients:

Spirits 100 grams, finger citron fruit 3,000 grams.

Pharmaceutical Process:

Wash the fruit clean and let it infuse in clear water till it gets soft. Cut it into cm cubes and let them dry. Put them into a jar, add the spirits and seal up the jar, stirring the mixture once every 5 days. Open the jar after 10 days and filtrate the mixture to remove the dregs.

Actions:

Soothes the liver, regulates the spleen, promotes digestion and dissolves sputum.

Indications:

Stagnation of the liver-qi, mental depression induced by the stagnancy of the spleen-qi and the stomach-qi, loss of appetite, fullness and pain in the chest and hypochondrium, nausea and vomiting, cough and abundant expectoration. Fingered citron fruit can also be used to dispel the effect of alcohol, so it kills two birds with one stone to dispel the effect of alcohol with the spirits medicated with fingered citron fruit because with the help of the spirits the medicine becomes more effective and sobers up a drunkard with little irritation.

Source:

Tonic recipes of Huiantang of Chengdu City in *Chinese Med-*

icated Dietetics, 1985, p. 185.

6. Wine of Aniseed

Ingredients:

Aniseed.

Pharmaceutical Process:

Let the seed soak in wine and drink it.

Indications:

Stomachache, swelling with bearing-down pain in one testis and pain in the chest or abdomen.

Source:

A Handbook of Family Dietetic Therapy, 1982, p. 154.

Put 15 grams of ground aniseed into a bag, let it soak in 500 grams of millet wine for 10 days and then take 15 ml. of it 3 times per day.

7. Spirit of Litchi Fruit

Ingredients:

5 litchi fruits, one cup of white spirits.

Pharmaceutical Process:

Boil the fruit in the spirit.

Indications:

Deficiency of *qi* and cold in the stomach.

Administration and Dosage:

3 times per day.

Source:

A Handbook of Family Dietectic Therapy, 1982, p. 103.

8. Spirit of Amomum Tsao-Ko

Ingredients:

Fruit of Amomum tsao-ko 10 grams, white spirit 250 grams,

dried orange peel and haw qs.

Pharmaceutical Process:

Let the herbs and fruit soak in the spirits for 7 days.

Indications:

Distention and pains in the gastric cavity and abdomen.

Administration and Dosage:

Oral administration.

Source:

Chinese Medicated Dietetics, 1985, p. 237.

9. Spirit of Walnuts

Ingredients:

Green walnuts 300 grams, white spirit 500 grams, syrup of monose 135ml.

Pharmaceutical Process:

Wash the walnuts clean and pound them to pieces. Put them into a bottle, add the spirits, seal up the bottle and keep it in scorching sunlight for 20 days till both the spirits and the walnuts turn black. Filtrate them and add the monose.

Indications:

Gastric and dodenal ulcer and gastritis.

Administration and Dosage:

10ml doses, twice per day, or take 10ml of it when there is a pain.

Source:

Intermediate Medical Periodical, *Encyclopedia of Chinese Dietetic Therapy*, 1988, p. 657.

10. Wine of Osmanthus Flowers

Ingredients:

Osmanthus flowers 60 grams, millet wine 500 grams.

Pharmaceutical Process:

Let the flowers soak in the wine for 15 days.

Actions:

Resolves sputum and dissipates blood stasis.

Indications:

Pains due to stagnated liver-*qi* and stomach-*qi*, belching and abdominal distention.

Administration and Dosage:

30ml doses, twice per day.

Source:

Family Manual of Flowers

11. Wine of Rose Flowers

Ingredients:

Rose flowers 30 grams, millet wine 500 grams.

Pharmaceutical Process:

Let the flowers soak in the wine for half a month.

Indications:

Pains due to the stagnated liver-*qi* and stomach-*qi*, menoxenia and leukorrhea.

Administration and Dosage:

20ml doses, twice per day.

Source:

Medicinal Herbs

12. Spirit of Cinnamon Bark

Ingredients:

Ground cinnamon bark 20 grams.

Pharmaceutical Process:

Let the bark soak in 1,000 grams of white spirit for half a month.

Indications:

Stomachache and abdominal pain of the type of deficiency and cold, dysmenorrhea.

Administration and Dosage:

10ml.

Source:

Materia Medica of Dietetic Therapy

13. Wine of Corianders

Ingredients:

Corianders 1,000 grams, grape wine.

Pharmaceutical Process:

Wash the corianders clean, cut them into segments and let them soak in 500ml of grape wine for 3 days. Then remove the corianders.

Indication:

Stomachache.

Administration and Dosage:

20ml or take it when ever there is pain.

Source:

1,100 *Folk Prescriptions of Dietetic Therapy*, 1992, p. 29.

14. Warming Spirit

Ingredients:

Cloves 6 grams, fingered citron fruit 10 grams, cinnamon bark 12 grams, galangal rhizome 4. 5 grams, seed of nutmeg 10 grams, amomum fruit 6 grams; fruit of Alpinia galanga, cinnamom twig, *Amomum cardamomum* 10 grams each; katsumadai seed 6 grams, root of Dahurian angelica 10 grams, rice fermented with red yeast 50 grams.

Actions:

Warms the middle-*jiao*, resolves dampness, regulates the stomach, dispels cold and alleviates pain.

Indications:

Pain in the gastric cavity, chest pain, vomiting, belching.

Administration and Dosage:

Oral administration, 10—20ml. doses, 1—3 times per day. Children under 3 take 2ml, children aged 3—6 2.5ml, children aged 6—10 3—4ml and children aged 10—15 5ml per dose.

Caution:

Pregnant women must not take it because it has a strong warming capacity which promotes blood circulation.

Source:

Practical Prepared Chinese Medicine, 1991, p. 540.

Section Five   Vomiting

1. Wine of Perilla Leaves and Orange Peel

Ingredients:

Dried perilla leaves 10 grams, dried orange peel 10 grams.

Pharmaceutical Process:

Decoct the ingredients in wine and water of equal quantity.

Indications:

Cold and vomiting.

Administration and Dosage:

Oral and separate administration.

Source:

Chinese Medicated Dietetics, 1985, p. 274.

2. Wine of Tangerine Peel

Ingredients:

Dried tangerine peel 60 grams, millet wine 1,000 grams.

Pharmaceutical Process:

Grind the peel and let it soak in the wine for 10 days.

Actions:

Regulates the flow of *qi* and whets the appetite.

Indications:

Vomiting, nausea, lack of appetite and abdominal distention.

Administration and Dosage:

30ml doses, twice per day.

Source:

Proved Recipes

Section Six   Indigestion

Anorexia of the stomach causes indigestion, so food stagnates in the stomach and intestines and that induces loss of appetite and a sensation of satiety.

1. Spirit of Orange Peel

Ingredients:

Dried orange peel 50 grams, white spirit 500 grams.

Pharmaceutical Process:

Let the peel soak in the spirit for 7 days.

Indications:

Indigestion and lack of appetite.

Administration and Dosage:

10—15ml 2 or 3 times per day.

Source：

 Chinese Medicated Dietetics, 1985, p. 242.

2. Spirit of Amomum Fruit

Ingredients：

 Amomum fruit 30 grams, white spirit 500 grams.

Pharmaceutical Process：

 Pound the fruit into pulp, wrap it up in clean gauze and let it soak in the spirits for 7 days.

Actions：

 Promotes digestion, regulates the stomach, keeps the adverse *qi* flowing downward and alleviates pain.

Indications：

 Indigestion and distention and pains in the gastric cavity and abdomen.

Administration：

 Oral administration after meal *q. s.*

Source：

 Chinese Medicated Dietetics, 1985, p. 236.

3. Wine of *Shenqu*

Ingredients：

 Shenqu (fermented mix of flour, bran, almonds, red beans, achene of Siberian cocklebur, *Artemisia apiacea*) 90 grams, millet wine 1,000 grams.

Pharmaceutical Process：

 Grind the mix and let it soak in the wine for 7 days.

Indications：

 Stagnation of food and indigestion.

Administration and Dosage：

42

30 gram doses, twice per day.

Source:

Zhaiyuanfang

4. Wine of Haws

Ingredients:

Haws and longan pulp 250 grams each; jujube fruit and brown sugar 30 grams each; millet wine 1,000 grams.

Pharmaceutical Process:

Let the ground fruit and sugar infue in the wine for 10 days.

Indications:

Retention of meat food in the stomach and indigestion, distention and fullness of the gastric cavity and abdomen.

Administration and Dosage:

20ml each time.

Source:

Medicinal Fruit

5. Wine of Green Plum

Ingredients:

Green plum 30 grams, yellow millet wine 100ml.

Pharmaceutical Process:

Soak the fruit in the wine in a china cup, put the cup into a larger container with water and heat it for 20 minutes.

Indications:

Lack of appetite, chronic indigestion and ascaris pain in the abdomen.

Administration and Dosage:

20ml doses while it is warm.

Source:

6. Wine of Astragalus Root

Ingredients:

Astragalus root 120 grams.

Pharmaceutical Process:

Grind the root and let it soak in 1,000 grams of millet wine for 7 days.

Indications:

Asthenia of the spleen and the stomach, lack of appetite, anorexia, palpitation, dyspnea, weakness of the limbs, general deficiency, hyperhydrosis, deficiency of *qi* and proctoptosis.

Administration and Dosage:

20ml doses, twice per day.

Source:

Prescriptions for Fmergencies

Section Seven   Hypochondriac Pain

Hypochondriac pain mainly refers to the pain in one side or both sides of the hypochondrium and is a common subjective clinical symptom.

1. Spirit of Nutgrass Flatsedge

Ingredients:

Prepared rhizome of nutgrass flatsedge 30 grams, white spirits 500 grams.

Pharmaceutical Process:

Let the rhizome soak in the spirit for 7 days.

Indications:

Stagnation of the liver-*qi*, hypochondriac pain and abdominal pain.

Administration and Dosage:

20ml doses, 3 or 4 times per day.

Source:

Chinese Medicated Dietetics, 1985, p. 243.

Section Eight   Diarrhea, Cholera and Dysentery

Diarrhea means too frequent emptying of the bowels and discharge of thin and watery excrement. Dysentery's major symptoms are abdominal pain, rectal tenesmus, and discharge of red and white or sanguinopurulent excrement. The symptoms of cholera are a sudden onset, vomiting, diarrhea and abdominal pain.

1. Wine of Chinese Chives

Ingredients:

Chinese chives.

Pharmaceutical Process:

Cut off the tips of the chives and mix a cup of wine with their juice.

Indications:

Dysentery and precordial pain.

Administration:

Take it while it is warm.

Source:

A Handbook of Family Dietetic Therapy, 1982, p. 11.

2. Wine of Galangal

Ingredients:

Galangal rhizome 70 grams, millet wine 200ml.

Pharmaceutical Process:

Parch the rhizome till it gets crisp and smells good, pound it to pieces, add the wine, and decoct them till they boil for the third or fourth time.

Indications:

Cholera, vomiting, dysentery and abdominal pain.

Administration and Dosage:

3 times per day.

Source:

Chinese Medicated Dietetics, 1985, p. 247.

3. Wine of Pig Pancreas

Ingredients:

A pig pancreas, 1,000 grams of limeless wine, 30 grams of sweet wormwood leaves and cassia bark respectively.

Pharmaceutical Process:

Cut the pancreas into small pieces, mix them with the wormwood leaves, warm the wine over a slow fire, and mix it with the minced pancreas and bark while it is still warm.

Actions:

Tonifies the five viscera and regulates the lung-*qi*.

Indications:

Deficiency caused by dysentery and cold, soreness and pain in the knees and tibia, stagnation of *qi* and blood stasis of women, weakness in the limbs, men's edema caused by deficiency and distention of the hypochondrium.

Administration and Dosage:

15ml in the morning, at noon and in the evening respectively.

Cautions:

Do not eat hot and greasy food while taking it.

Source:

A Handbook of Family Dietetic Therapy, 1982, p. 510.

4. Wine of Duck Blood

Ingredients:

Live duck.

Pharmaceutical Process:

Slaughter the duck and pour its blood to boiling wine and drink the mixture.

Actions:

Tonifies the blood and removes toxic substances.

Indications:

Hematemesis due to internal injury caused by overstrain, dysentery.

Administration and Dosage:

3 times per day.

Source:

Chinese Dietetic Therapy, p. 172.

Remarks:

It can also be used to treat tidal fever during menstruation and also lack of appetite.

A Handbook of Family Dietetic Therapy, 1982, p. 205.

Section Nine   Constipation

Constipation means having difficulty in emptying bowels and is a common symptom which often occurs in various kinds of acute and chronic diseases, especially the diseases of postpartum women and the elderly.

1. Wine of Hemp Seed

Ingredients:

Hemp seed 500 grams.

Pharmaceutical Process:

Grind the seeds and let them soak in 1,000 grams of millet wine for 7 days.

Actions:

Loosens the bowels and relieves constipation.

Indications:

Senile or postpartum impairment of body fluids, deficiency of blood and constipation.

Administration and Dosage:

30ml doses, twice per day.

Source:

Prescriptions for Emergencies

2. Wine of Peach Buds

Ingredients:

Peach buds 30 grams.

Pharmaceutical Process:

Grind the buds and let them soak in 500 grams of millet wine for 7 days.

Indication:

Constipation.

Administration and Dosage:

30ml doses, twice per day.

Source:

Prescriptions for Emergencies

3. Wine of Peach Kernels

Ingredients:

Peach kernels 60 grams.

Pharmaceutical Process:

Grind the kernels and let them soak in 1,000 grams of millet wine for 10 days.

Actions:

Loosens the bowels and relieves constipation.

Indications:

Postpartum deficiency of blood and constipation.

Administration and Dosage:

30 gram doses, twice a day.

Source:

Medicinal Fruit.

Section Ten   Arthralgia Syndrome

Arthralgia syndrome is caused by exogenous pathogenic factors like wind, cold, dampness and heat, etc. , which induce blockage of channels and collaterals and hinder the circulation of blood and *qi*. Its major clinical symptoms are myalgia, arthralgia, numbness, difficulty in stretching the limbs freely and even arthrocele and joint cauma. Clinically, it is a lingering disease and is similar to rheumatic arthritis, rheumatoid arthritis and gout in modern medicine.

1. Rheumatic Ostealgia Spirit No. 1

Ingredients:

Dried aerial parts of *Erodium stephanianum* 10,000 grams; rhizome of Chinese atractylodes 5,000 grams; *Phryma lep-*

tostachya var. asiatica 5,000 grams; cocklebur leaves 2,500 grams; dahuo 2,500 grams; bark of cork tree 2,500 grams; root of Chinese climatis 5,000 grams; *Ampelopsis aconitifolia Bge.* 5,000 grams; wild aconite root 250 grams; ledebouriella root 2,500 grams.

Pharmaceutical Process:

Decoct the bark of a cork tree for an hour, then add the other herbs and water to submerge them 2 *cun*. Decoct them till one-third of the water is left, filtrate them, and decoct them again in the same way. Remove the dregs, mix the two extracts, boil down the mixture to 3,000—3,500 grams, add 3,000 grams of sugar and 20,000 grams of white spirits and mix them well. The quantities of the ingredients can be reduced in the above proportions.

Actions:

Dispels wind, removes dampness, relieves inflammation and alleviates pains.

Indications:

Pains in the waist and lower extremities induced by wind-cold and numbness of muscles and joints.

Administration and Dosage:

Oral administration, 15—20ml doses, 2—3 times per day.

Storage:

Keep it airtight and away from light.

Source:

Office of the Exhibition of Chinese Medicinal Herbs and New Therapy of Heilongjiang Province, *Selection of the Materials of the National Exhibition of Chinese Medicinal Herbs and New Therapy*.

2. Rheumatic Ostealgia Spirit No. 2

Ingredients:

Rhizome of *Toddalia asiatica Lam.* 100 grams, sargentgloryvine 100 grams, cibot rhizome 100 grams, rhizome of giant knotweed 100 grams, *Schefflera arboricola* 100 grams, *Piper boehmeriaefolium Wall.* 100 grams, alangium root 100 grams.

Pharmaceutical Process:

Cut the herbs into small pieces and increase their volume to 2,000ml by adding spirits. Let them soak for a month, filtrate the infusion, and again increase the volume of the filtrate to 2,000ml by spirits.

Actions:

Dispels wind and dampness and removes the obstruction in the channels and collaterals to promote blood circulation.

Indications:

Traumatic injury and rheumatic arthritis.

Administration and Dosage:

Oral administration, 10ml doses, 3 times per day.

Storage:

Keep it airtight in a dark place.

Source:

Pharmaceutical Factory of Unit 35215 of the Chinese People's Liberation Army, *Selection of Rural Prescriptions of Chinese Medicinal Herbs*, 1976, p. 26.

3. Rheumatic Ostealgia Spirit No. 3

Ingredients:

Spatholobus stem 150 grams, leafy stem of Chinese starjasmine 150 grams, rhizome of slender acanthopanax 50 grams, fruit of Chinese flowering quince 100 grams, loranthus mulberry mistletoe 150 grams, spirits *q. s.*, futokadsura stem 150 grams.

Pharmaceutical Process:

Cut the herbs into thin slices and make 1,500 grams of medicated spirit of them with the method of extraction by infusion in cool spirits (See Chapter Two).

Actions:

Dispels dampness, relieves the rigidity of the muscles and tendons and removes the obstruction in the channels and collaterals.

Indications:

Rheumatic arthritis and arthralgia.

Administration and Dosage:

Oral administration, once or twice per day and 25—50 grams each time.

Source:

Pharmaceutical Techniques of Chinese Herbal Medicine of Zhejiang Province, ed. Station of Medicinal Inspection of Zhejiang Province et al, 1976, p. 222.

4. Wine of *Erycibe Obtusifolia*

Ingredients:

Erycibe obtusifolia 200 grams.

Pharmaceutical Process:

Cut the ingredient into small pieces, steam them for half an hour and add a *proper quantity* of millet wine containing 50% alcohol. Let them soak for 15 days, filtrate them and get 1,000 grams of extract.

Indication:

Rheumatic pains in the waist and lower extremities.

Administration and Dosage:

Oral administration, 15—20ml doses, twice per day.

Source:

Selection of Rural Prescriptions of Chinese Medicinal Herbs, ed. Station of Medicinal Inspection of Guangzhou City, 1971, p. 132.

5. Wine of *Sarcandra Glabra Nakai*

Ingredients:

Scarcandra glabra Nakai 45 grams, hongyuyan 45 grams. *Sectionhenocissus heterophylla Merr.* 30 grams, shandafeng 30 grams.

Pharmaceutical Process:

Let the herbs soak in 2,500 grams of wine containing 55% alcohol for 15 days. Remove the settled dregs and use the clear extract for treatment.

Actions:

Dispels cold and removes dampness.

Indication:

Rheumatic arthritis.

Administration and Dosage:

Oral administration (if the patient can drink wine and has no contraindications), 20ml doses, twice per day; 2,000ml constitute a course of treatment.

Source:

Chinese Medicinal Herbs, 1971, p. 37.

6. Spirit for Arthritis

Ingredients:

Sichuan aconite root 6 grams, Chinese wolfberry fruit 9 grams, safflower 6 grams, eucommia bark 9 grams, wild aconite root 6 grams, Chinese angelica root 6 grams, chaenomeles fruit 9 grams, black-tail snake 9 grams, achyranthes root 9 grams, pilose asiabell root 6 grams.

Pharmaceutical Process:

Let the herbs soak in 500 grams of white spirits containing 60 grams of alcohol for a week.

Actions:

Promotes blood circulation, dispels wind, and strengthens the bones and muscles.

Indication:

Rheumatic arthritis.

Administration and Dosage:

Oral administration, 15ml doses, 3 times per day.

Source:

Selection of the Prescriptions of Chinese Medicinal Herbs, ed. Beijing Medical College *et al*, 1971, p. 85.

7. Spirit of *Polygonum Cuspidatum*

Ingredients:

Root of *Polygonum cuspidatum* 500 grams, root of *Caragana sinica* 500 grams.

Pharmaceutical Process:

Wash the herbs clean, cut them into thin slices, dry them and submerge them in water in a pot. Decoct them for an hour, stirring them frequently; filtrate the decoction, decoct the herbs again in the same way and mix the filtrated decoctions. Boil down the mixture over a slow fire to 200 grams or so, add 700ml of white spirit when it cools somewhat, mix them so that they cannot congeal, then pour the mixture into a clean bottle when it cools down. Keep it static for a night, remove the settled dregs by filtration, add white spirit again to increase the quantity of the extract to 1,000 grams and add 1 gram of saccharin dissolved in a little boiled water. Mix them and seal the mixture in a clean, dry brown glass bottle.

Actions:

Eliminates dampness and heat, dissipates blood stasis and and promotes blood circulation.

Indications:

Arthralgia and rheumatic arthritis.

Administration and Dosage:

Oral administration, 10ml doses, three times per day.

Storage:

Keep it airtight in a dark and cool place.

Source:

In stitute of Medical Industry of Shanghai, *Medical Industry*, 1971, Issue 5, p. 34.

8. Spirit of Futokadsura

Ingredients:

Futokadsura stem 125 grams, inflorescence of *Echinops latifolius Tausch* 125 grams.

Pharmaceutical Process:

Let the herbs soak in some white spirits containing 40—60% alcohol and obtain 1,000ml of extract from them with the method of extraction by infusion in Chapter Two.

Actions:

Dispels wind and dampness, and removes the obstruciton in the channels to relieve pain.

Indications:

Rheumatic arthritis, bronchial asthma and bronchitis.

Administration and Dosage:

Oral administration, 10ml doses before breakfast and supper. Do not heat it before drinking it.

Source:

Rural Pharmaceutical Techniques of Chinese Herbal Medicine, ed. Station of Medicinal Inspection of Guangzhou City, 1971, p. 115.

9. Spirit of Alangium

Ingredients:

Chinese alangium root.

Pharmaceutical Process:

Wash the root clean and cut it into thin slices. Let them soak in white spirits (1 : 3) for 20 days, stirring them every other day and sealing up the container immediately. Remove the settled dregs and filtrate the liquid.

Actions:

Dispels wind and dampness and relaxes muscles and tendons and promotes the flow of blood and *qi* in the channels and collaterals.

Indication:

Chronic rheumatic arthritis.

Administration and Dosage:

Oral administration, 10ml doses, 2 or 3 times per day.

Source:

Hospital of Jiukou District of Zhongxiang Country, Hubei
Province, *New Medicine*, Issue 8, 1972, p. 33.

10. Wine of Schisandra

Ingredients:

Rhizome of schisandra with small flowers 60 grams.

Pharmaceutical Process:

Let the rhizome soak in 500 grams of wine for 5—7 days.

Actions:

Dispels wind and dampness and promotes the flow of *qi* to
alleviate pain.

Indications:

Rheumatic ostealgia and traumatic injury.

Administration and Dosage:

Oral administration, 10 ml. doses, 3 times per day.

Source:

Selection of Chinese Medicinal Herbs, Vol. One, 1973, p.
93.

11. Instant Extract of Chaenomeles Fruit

Ingredients:

Chaenomeles fruit 18,250 grams, mulberry branches 25,000
grams, rhizome of *Ligusticum wallichii* 6,250 grams, loranthus
mulberry mistletoe 16,250 grams, gastrodia tuber 6,250 grams,
Chinese angelica root 12,500 grams, teasel root 12,500 grams,
spikenard root 6,250 grams, safflower 12,500 grams, achyranthes root 18,750 grams, unprepared fragrant solomonseal rhizome 31,250 grams, prepared cibot rhizome, alcohol with a concentration of 50% *q. s.*, cane sugar *q. s.*

Pharmaceutical Process:

Pound all the herbs to pieces except the safflower and sift them with a sieve. The diameter of each of its meshes should be 1 centimeter. Add the safflower, mix them well, wet them with some of the alcohol and put the mixture into a percolator. Percolate it according to the normal procedure, obtain the percolate and retrieve the alcohol in a decompressor till the percolate gets sticky; then add some sugar powder, mix well, make the mixture into granules, dry them, and wrap them in plastic film bags.

The medicine consists of dry and light yellow granules with a slightly sweet taste. Each of the bags has 50 grams of granules with potency equal to 500 grams of medicated spirit.

Actions:

Dispels wind and cold, promotes the circulation of blood and strengthens the muscles and tendons and bones.

Indications:

Cold, wind, dampness, contracture of the muscles and blood vessels and pains in the limbs.

Administration and Dosage:

Dissolve the granules of each bag in 500 grams of white spirits and drink no more than 200 grams of it each time.

Source:

No. 2 Pharmaceutical Factory of Chinese Medicine of Hanzhou, Zhejiang Province, *Bulletin of Science and Technology*, 1973, Issue 9.

12. Rheumatism Spirit No. 1

Ingredients:

Rhizome of Chinese atractylodes 6,000 grams, sorghum

rootlets and foliferous stem and branch of *Loranthus parasiticus* 6,000 grams each, fruit of Chinese flowering quince and achyranthus root 6,000 grams each, egg plant root 6,000 grams, eucommia bark.

Pharmaceutical Process:

Let the herbs soak in 150,000 grams of white spirit for more than a month, stirring them frequently, filtrate them and use the clear extract for treatment.

Actions:

Dispels wind-dampness, strengthens the waist and the knees and alleviates pain.

Indication:

Pain caused by rheumatic arthritis.

Administration and Dosage:

10ml per day.

Source:

Common Prescriptions of Traditonal Chinese Medicine and Western Medicine and Ways to Make Them Up, ed. Pharmaceutical Factory of the No. 1 People's Hospital of Chengdu City, 1973

13. Rheumatism Spirit No. 2

Ingredients:

Babaili 30 grams, rhizome of *Scopolia acutangula C.* 15 grams, peppermint, camphoz and borneol *q. s.* each.

Pharmaceutical Process:

Let the ingredients soak in 500 grams of spirits for 7 days.

Indications:

Rheumatic arthritis and traumatic injury.

Administration and Dosage:

Smear it on the affected part several times per day.

Caution:

Do not drink it because it is highly toxic.

Source:

Station of Prevention and Treatment of Diseases of Guilin Prefecture, Guangxi, *Selection of the Materials of the National Exhibition of Chinese Medicinal Herbs and New Therapy*, 1972, p. 200.

14. Rheumatism Spirit No. 3

Ingredients:

Prepared Sichuan aconite root 15 grams, prepared fleece-flower root 15 grams, prepared wild aconite root 6 grams, *Echinops latifolius Tausch* 9 grams, rhizome of *Homalomena occulata* 9 grams, white spirits 500 grams.

Pharmaceutical Process:

Let the herbs soak in the spirit airtight for 48 hours and filtrate them.

Actions:

Dispels wind and cold, promotes the circulation of blood and alleviates pain.

Indications:

Rheumatic arthritis, rheumatoid arthritis and pains in the waist and lower extremities.

Administration and Dosage:

Oral administration, 5-19ml doses, 3 times per day.

Source:

Collection of Chinese Medicinal Herbs, vol. 1, 1973, p. 308.

15. Rheumatism Spirit No. 4

Ingredients:

Sargentgloryvine 300 grams, prepared Sichuan aconite root 90 grams, prepared wild aconite root 90 grams, safflower 90 grams, black plum 90 grams, honeysuckle flowers 150 grams, licorice root 150 grams, white spiritS 500 grams.

Pharmaceutical Process:

Prepare the herbs and put them into a bottle. Warm up the spirit, pour it into the bottle and mix the ingredients well. Seal up the bottle, let the ingredients soak for 7 days and use the filtrate for treatment.

Actions:

Dispels wind, removes obstruction in the channels and collaterals to promote blood circulation and relaxes the muscles and tendons.

Indication:

Rheumatic arthritis.

Administration and Dosage:

5—10ml doses, 2 or 3 times per day; 7 days constitute a course of treatment.

Source:

Selected Materials of the Combination of Chinese and Western Medicine, ed. Military Medical School of Beijing Military Region, 1974, p. 160.

16. Rheumatism Spirit No. 5

Ingredients:

Mulberry bark, *Aster tataricus L. f.*, licorice root, *Ampelopsis aconitifolia Bge.*, ledebouriella root, fruit of Chinese flowering quince, rhizome of heracleum, prepared Sichuan aconite root, *Schizophragma intergrifolium Oliv.*, sargentgloryvine, rhizome of Chinese atractylodes (parched with bran), Chinese photinia, rhizome of cyathula, fruit of *Poncirus trifoliata* (parched with bran), ephedra twig, large-leaved gentian, eucommia bark (parched in salt water), cibot rhizome, teasel root, dried ginger, white eggplant root, root of *Asarum heterotropoides mandshuricum*, prepared rhizome of rehmannice, epimedium, fresh twig and leaf of oriental arborvitae (cut into segments), fresh and barked root of *Taxus cuspidata Sieb. et Zucc.*, spirits.

Actions:

Dispels wind and dampness, warms the channels to promote the flow of *qi*.

Indications:

Arthralgia, whose clinical symptoms are wandering pains in the joints, difficulty in stretching the limbs, thin, white and moist fur on the tongue, floating pulse, fixed sharp pains in the limbs that lessen when it is hot and worsen when it is cold, joint rigidity, tense and forceful pulse, numbness of the skin and muscles, sensation of heaviness in the hands and feet, floating, thready and soft pulse.

Administration and Dosage:

Oral administration 10—15ml doses, 2 or 3 times per day for adults.

Cautions:

Those who have hyperactivity of fire due to the deficiency of *yin* should be cautious in taking it and do not take in medicine containing pinellia, Trichosanthes kirilowi, hyacinth bletilla, ampelopsis and *Bulbus fritillariae* while taking the spirit.

Source:

Medicinal Criteria of Hunan Province, (1982) in *Basic Prescriptions of Chinese Medicine of China*, vol. 1, 1988, p. 63.

17. Rheumatism Spirit No. 6

Ingredients:

Honeysuckle, black plum, wild aconite root, Sichuan aconite root, licorice root and halite 6 grams each; safflower, black plum, wild aconite root, Sichuan aconite root and licorice root 9 grams each.

Pharmaceutical Process:

Let the first 6 ingredients soak in 500 grams of 60% proof spirit for 21 days for male patients; let the remaining ingredients soak in 500 grams of spirits for 7 days for female patients.

Indications:

Rheumatic arthritis and rheumatoid arthritis.

Administration and Dosage:

5ml dosee, 3 times per day.

Source:

The People's Hospital of Xinjin County of Luda City, Liaoning Province, *Selection of the Materials of the National Exhibition of Chinese Medicinal Herbs and New Therapy*, 1972, p. 196.

18. *Changning* Rheumatism Spirit

Ingredients:

Chinese angelica root 120 grams, glabrous greenbrier rhizome 90 grams, ledebouriella root 60 grams, rehmannia root 120 grams, root of Chinese climatis 90 grams, tetrandra root 60 grams, safflower 60 grams, Chinese flowering quince 30 grams.

Pharmaceutical Process:

Let the herbs soak in sorghum spirit containing 60% alcohol for 3 weeks, and filtrate them to obtain clear filtrate. Decoct the dregs, remove the dregs by filtration to obtain clear filtrate, and add 500 grams of cobra, Pallas pit viper and *Dinodon rufuzonatum* each (all live) Soak in 1,000 grams of spirit for 3 weeks. Mix the spirits in equal quantities, finally mixing the medicated and filtrated spirit, the filtrated decoction and the mixed snake spirits.

Actions:

Dispels wind and dampness, promotes the circulation of blood and alleviates pain.

Indication:

Rheumatoid arthritis.

Administration and Dosage:

Oral administration, 10ml doses, 3 times per day.

Source:

Journal of New Pharmacy, 1973, Issue 5, p. 23.

19. Rheumatism Spirit of *Dendropanax Chevalieri Merr*

Ingredients:

root of *Dendropanax chevalieri Merr.* 60 grams, rhizome of cyathula 12 grams, alangium root 30 grams, *Uncaria rhynchophylla* 12 grams, sargentgloryvine 18 grams, Cherokee rose hips 18 grams, root of red-rooted saliva 18 grams, white spirits 1,000 grams, cinnamom twig 12 grams, brown sugar 60 grams.

Pharmaceutical Process:

Cut the root of *Dendropanax chevalieri Merr.*, the alagium root and the Cherokee rosehips into slices and submerge them in water. Decoct them twice, bringing them to a boil and continue decocting them for 3—4 hours each time; then filtrate them and concentrate the filtrate into thick liquid. Cut the other herbs into slices, let them soak in hot spirit for a month, remove the dregs, filtrate them to obtain clear filtrate and mix the thick liquid, the filtrate and the sugar, which should be made into syrup before use. Keep the mixture static to settle it, filtrate it with a cloth and pour it into bottles.

Actions:

Dispels wind-dampness, removes obstruction in the channels and collaterals and relieves ankylosis.

Indications:

Rheumatic orthritis, traumatic injury, hemiparalysis, sprain and contusion.

Administration and Dosage:

Oral administration, 15 gram doses, 2 or 3 times per day.

Source:

Pharmacy, ed. Jiangxi Pharmaceutical School, 1973,

20. Spirit of Mountain Creeper

Ingredients:

Fresh mountain creeper leaves 3,500 grams, two live male crabs, four live ground beetles, 500 grams of white spirit.

Pharmaceutical Process:

Wash the leaves clean and mince them. Let them and the crabs and beetles soak in the spirit for a week.

Actions:

Promotes blood circulation and dispels dampness.

Indication:

Rheumatic arthritis.

Administration and Dosage:

15ml in the morning and the evening respectively.

Source:

Hubei Science and Technology, 1973, Issue 1, p. 77.

21. Analgesic Spirit

Ingredients:

Sichuan aconite root 30 grams, wild aconite rhizome 30 grams, pseudo-ginseng 15 grams, vomiting nuts 15 grams.

Pharmaceutical Process:

Wash the aconite rhizomes clean, cut them into slices and dry them in sunlight. Decoct them in 250 grams of honey, remove the fuzz of the vomiting nuts and fry them in plant oil. Pound the pseudo-ginseng to pieces, add water and decoct it twice. Add 1,000ml of water and concentrate the decoction to 300ml the first time; add 1,000ml of water and concentrate the decoction to 200ml the second time. The extracts obtained will thus amount to 500ml. Finally, add 500ml of ordinary white spirit.

Actions:

Dispels wind, promotes blood circulation, relaxes muscles and tendons and activates the channels and collaterals.

Indications:

Chronic pains in the waist and lower extremities.

Administration and Dosage:

Oral administration, 10ml doses, 3 times per day; 10 days constitute a course of treatment.

Source:

Jingzhou Hygiene, 1973, Issue 1, p. 30.

22. Arthritis Spirit

Ingredients:

Erycibe obtusifolia 19,200 grams, root of Dahurian angelica 16,000 grams, rhizome of slender acanthopanax 12,000 grams, ephedra twig 3,200 grams, sweet wormwood seed 1,600 grams, Chinese angelica root 1,000 grams, cinnamon twigs 1,600 grams, aniseeds 1,200 grams, rhizome of Ligusticum Chuanxiong 1,000 grams, root of Chinese climatis 1,600 grams, tetrandra root 1,200 grams, Fujian cape jasmine 1,000 grams, notopterygium root 1,200 grams, rhizome of heracleum 1,200 grams, white spirits (50% alcohol) 19,2001 grams.

Pharmaceutical Process:

Mix all the herbs well and add the spirits. Let them soak in a sealed container for 45 days in autumn or summer or 60 days in spring or winter. Filtrate them to obtain clear liquid, press the dregs to obtain extract, then mix the filtrate and the extract. Keep the mixture static for 4 days and filtrate it.

Actions:

Dispels wind and cold, removes obstruction in the channels and collaterals to alleviate pain.

Indications:

Paralysis due to wind-cold-dampness, numbness of the limbs, arthralgia and myalgia, lassitude in the loin and legs and wound dehiscence.

Administration and Dosage:

Oral administration, 25 grams doses, 3 times per day.

Source:

Criteria of Medicine of Shanghai City, 1974, p. 44.

23. Rheumatic Arthritis Spirit

Ingredients:

Rhizome of cyathula 90 grams, root of ledebouriella 120 grams, Chinese flowering quince fruit 60 grams, wild aconite root 90 grams (prepared in the water of licorice root and honesuckle flowers), root of Chinese climatis 60 grams, cinnamom twigs 90 grams, rhizome of *Dioscorea hypoclauca Palib.* 150 grams, rhizome of Ligusticum Chuanxiong 150 grams, nodular branch of pine 150 grams, Chinese angelica root 150 grams, spatholobus stem 120 grams, Japanese yam rhizome 240 grams, rhizome of Chinese atractylodes 150 grams, root of herbaceous peony 150 grams, black-tail snake (prepared in spirits) 150 grams, ginseng 120 grams, fingered citron fruit 150 grams, herb of common heron's bill 240 grams, licorice root 120 grams, rice fermented with red yeast 240 grams, rhizome of slender acanthopanax 240 grams, noterpterygium root 90 grams, rhizome of heracleum 240 grams, brown sugar 3,000 grams, baimi 5,000 grams.

Pharmaceutical Process:

Wash the ingredients clean and put them into a clean container. Add 2,500 grams, 1,500 grams and 1,000 grams of white spirits containing 45% alcohol and 8 *liang* of rice fermented with red yeast separately. Wait an interval of half an hour after the ingredients boil before obtaining the extract each time. Press the dregs, mix the extract with those previously obtained and put the mixture into a jar. Keep it static for a month and filtrate it.

Actions:

Dispels wind-cold-dampness, promotes blood circulation and alleviates pain.

Indications:

Arthralgia, aching pains in the shoulders and the back and numbness of the extremities.

Administration and Dosage:

Oral administration, twice per day and 15—30 grams each time.

Caution:

Pregnant women must not take it.

Source:

Criteria of Prepared Chinese Medicine of Beijing City, 1974, Vol. 2

24. Spirit of Giant Knotweed

Ingredients:

Rhizome of giant knotweed.

Pharmaceutical Process:

Cut the rhizome into slices, let them soak in white spirits (250 : 750) and seal up the container. Open it half a month later, add a little brown sugar.

Actions:

Dispels heat and dampness, removes the obstruction in the channels and collaterals to promote blood circulation and dissipates blood stasis.

Indication:

Arthritis.

Administration and Dosage:

Oral administration, twice per day and 5 *qian* each time for adults.

Cautions:

Women who have menorrhagia must not take it during menstrual period; those allergic to spirits (e. g. skin rash and itching, etc.) should not take it, or they can take a smaller dose; those who have chronic hepatitis or who are not fit to drink spirits must not take it.

Source:

Journal of New Pharmaceatics, 1974, Issue 7, p. 32.

25. Wine of *Pterospermum Heterophyllum Hance*

Ingredients:

Leaves of *Pterospermum heterophyllum Hance* 1,500 grams, rhizome of slender acanthopanax 1,500 grams, bark of *Cinnamomum burmannii Bl.* 1,500 grams, fleece-flower root 1,500 grams, rhizome of *Moghania philippinensis Li.* 1,500 grams, dried tangerine peel 1,000 grams, Chinese angelica root 1,500 grams, prepared Sichuan aconite root 1,000 grams, achyranthes root 1,000 grams.

Pharmaceutical Process:

Wash the ingredients clean, cut them into slices and put them into an enamel mug. Add 50,000 grams of wine of cane sugar containing 50—60% alcohol, seal up the mug and let the herbs soak for 2—3 weeks (a few days shorter in summer and a few days longer in winter). Filtrate them and use the clear filtrate for treatment.

Actions:

Dispels wind-dampness, strengthens the muscles and tendons and alleviates pain.

Indications:

Lumbar muscle strain, sprain and rheumatoid spondilitis.

Administration and Dosage:

Oral administration, twice per day and 25 grams for addults.

Source:

Guangxi Hygiene, 1975, Issue 2, p. 47.

26. Paralysis Spirit

Ingredients:

Rhizome of *Scopolia sinensis Hemsl* 1,000 grams, cymose buckwheat rhizome 2,000 grams, root of Chinese climatis 2,500 grams, hairy birthwort rhizome 2,500 grams, common St. Paulswort 4,000 grams, European verbena 3,000 grams, jinjier 2,000 grams.

Pharmaceutical Process:

Grind the herbs and let them soak in 125,000 grams of spirit for more than 3 weeks, stirring them at intervals. Extract the clear part of the infusion, press the dregs and filtrate them.

Actions:

Dispels wind-dampness and heat and relieves inflammation.

Indications:

Rheumatic paralysis and pain.

Administration and dosage:

Oral administration, 5—10ml doses, 3 times per day.

Source:

Pharmacopoeia of Chinese Herbal Medicine, ed. Public Health Bureau of Macheng County, Hubei Province, 1975, p. 88—89.

27. Spirit of Ledebouriella

Ingredients:

Ledebouriella root 1,000 grams, eucommia bark (parched) 1,500 grams, large-leaved gentian 1,000 grams, rhizome of cyathula 1,000 grams, silkworm excrement 1,000 grams, safflower 500 grams, rhizome of *Dioscorea hypoclauca Palib.* 1,000 grams, root of egg plant 2,000 grams, noterpterygium root 500 grams, freshwater turtle shell (prepared) 500 grams, dried orange peel 500 grams, rhizome of large-headed atractylodes (parched) 1,000 grams, cocklebur fruit 1,000 grams, Chinese wolfberry fruit 2,000 grams, Chinese angelica root 1,000 grams, sugar 40,000 grams.

Pharmaceutical Process:

Wash the ingredients, then grind the ingredients from the ledebouriella root to the wolfberyy fruit into small pieces and pulverize the sugar. Percolate the ground ingredients with 25% proof alcohol at five times the quantity of the ingredients, retrieve the alcohol of the percolate, and concentrate the percolate to 4,000 grams of thick extract. Mix it well with the powdered sugar, sift the mixture with a sieve with 14—16 meshes and make it into granules. Dry them by airing or by low temperature desiccation, spray flavouring essence over them, seal them up in a pail, then pack them separately 2 days later into bags which can hold 50 grams of medicine each (about 350 bags in all).

Actions:

Dispels wind and promotes blood circulation.

Indications:

Soreness and pains in the extremities and arthralgia due to wind-cold and lassitude of the loins and the knees.

Administration and Dosage:

Dissolve the granules of each bag in 800 grams of spirit and drink no more than 200 grams each time.

Cautions:

Hypertention patients and pregnant women must not take it.

Source:

A Handbook of Chinese Medicinal Prescriptions, ed. Research Institute of Chinese Medicine, 1975, p. 685.

28. Lumbago Spirit

Ingredients:

Eucommia bark 25 grams, fruit of *Psoralea corylifolia* 15 grams, deglued antler powder 15 grams.

Pharmaceutical Process:

Grind the ingredients into small pieces, let them infuse in 500 grams of spirits and filtrate them.

Indications:

Rheumatic lumbago and senile lumbago.

Administration and Dosage:

Oral administration, 20ml doses, twice per day in the morning and the evening. 7 days constitute a course of treatment.

Source:

Pharmacopoeia of Chinese Herbal Medicine, ed. Public Health Bureau of Macheng County, Hubei Province, 1975, p. 89.

29. Anti-Rheumatism Spirit No. 1

Ingredients:

Rhizome of slender acanthopanax 20 grams, twigs of ephedra 20 grams, Sichuan aconite root (prepared) 20 grams, licorice root 20 grams, black plum 20 grams, wild aconite root (prepared) 20 grams, fruit of Chinese flowering quince 20 grams, alcohol (60%, diluted to 1,000 grams), safflower 20 grams.

Pharmaceutical Process:

Let the herbs soak in the alcohol for 10 days. Then filtrate the infusion and keep the filtrate static for 24 hours before filtrating it again. 1ml of the medicated alcohol is equal to 160mg of the herbs in potency.

Actions:

Relaxes the muscles and tendons and dispels wind and dampness.

Indication:

Rheumatic arthritis.

Administration and Dosage:

Oral administration, 5—10ml doses, 3 times per day.

Source:

Pharmacopoeia of Rural Prescritions of Chinese Herbal Medicine, ed. Station of Medicinal Inspection of the Scientific and Technical Commission of Honghe Prefecture, Yunnan Province, 1976, p. 24.

30. Anti-Rheumatism Spirit No. 2

Ingredients:

Phryma leptostachya var. asiatica (whole plant), rhizome of *Myrsine africana L.*, rhizome of dioamacao, *fanbeihong*, rhizome of *manshanxiang*, Chinese yam and rhizome of *lycopodium clavatum L.* 15 grams each; rhizome of alangium, astragalus root 12 grams each; Piper kadsura Ohwi, white-flowered *Gynura bodinieri Levl.* root 9 grams each; root bark of eucommia 3 grams.

Pharmaceutical Process:

Let the herbs soak in 1,000 grams of spirits for 3 days.

Indications:

Rheumatic arthritis and rheumatoid arthritis.

Administration and Dosage:

5—15ml doses 2 or 3 times per day. Replenish the medicated spirit with the quantity equal to that taken each day.

Cautions:

Do not eat bean products, mutton, sour or cold food while taking the spirit and pregnant women must not take it.

Source:

Hospital of Yangguang Commune of Tonghai County, Yunnan Province, *Selection of the Materials of the National Exhibition of Chinese Medicinal Herbs and New Therapy*, 1972, p. 204.

31. Spirit of Long-Noded Pit Viper

Ingredients:

Long-noded pit viper 12 grams, noterpterygium root 6 grams, safflower 15 grams, ledebourriella root 3 grams, rhizome of elevated gastrodia 6 grams, rhizome of slender acanthopanax 6 grams, sugar 150 grams, large-leaved gentian 6 grams.

Pharmaceutical Process:

Grind the ingredients to very small pieces and percolate them with 1,000 grams of spirits.

Actions:

Dispels dampness and removes the obstruction in the channels and collaterals.

Indications:

Rheumatic or rheumatoid arthritis, arthralgia, etc.

Administration and Dosage:

Oral administration, no more than 100 gram doses, twice per

day.

Source:

Pharmaceutical Techniques of Chinese Herbal Medicine of Zhejiang Province,ed. Station of Medicinal Inspection of Zhejiang Province *et al*, 1976, p. 222.

32. Spirit of Tiger Bone

Ingredients:

Tiger bone, noterpterygium, cinnamon twig, eucommia bark, Sichuan aconite rhizome (prepared), fruit of Chinese flowering quince, rhizome of heracleum, ephedra twig, psoralea fruit, rhizome of wild fruit (prepared), rhizome of Chinese atractylodes, rhizome of slender acanthopanax, Chinese angelica root, root of Chinese climatis, madder, *Poria coccos*, safflower, teasel root, fleece-flower root, bark of Chinese cassia tree, rhizome of Ligusticum Chuanxiong, large-leaved gentian, *Dioscorea hypoglauce*, licorice root, dried orange peel, eggplant root, antler, rhizome of cyathula, sugar, spirits.

Actions:

Dispels wind and dampness and promotes blood circulation to relieve pain.

Indications:

Paralysis due to wind-cold-dampness. Symptoms are arthralgia, wandering or static pain, swelling pains and numbness in the joints of the extremities, lassitude of the loins and knees and soft, floating pulse.

Administration and Dosage:

Oral administration, 15ml doses, twice per day for adults.

Cautions:

76

Do not take medicine containing pinellia, *Trichosanthes kirilowi*, hyacinth bletilla and ampelopsis while taking the spirits; pregnant women must not take it.

Source:

Medicinal Criteria of Jiangxi Province, 1982, in Basic Prescriptions of Chinese Medicine of China, 1988, P. 44

33. Spirit of Panther Bone

Ingredients:

Panther bone (crisped), teasel root, fruit of Chinese flowering quince, rhizome of acanthopanax, Chinese angelica root, twig of mulberry, rhizome of Ligusticum Chuanxiong, ledebouriella root, gastrodia tuber, rhizome of cyathula, safflower, rhizome of polygonatum, large-leaved gentian, white egg plant root, rock candy, 60% proof spirits.

Actions:

Dispels wind, dampness and cold to relieve pain.

Indications:

Paralysis (arthralgia, rigidity and muscle and tendon spasm, numbness of the extremities, pale tongue with thin, white fur and soft, floating pulse) and facial palsy (distortion of eyes and mouth caused by the invasion of pathogenic wind into the collaterals).

Administration and Dosage:

Oral administration, 10—15ml doses, twice per day for adults.

Cautions:

Patients who have deficiency of *yin* and internal heat with a a fever due to cold must not take it.

Source:

Medicinal Criteria of Jiangsu Province, (1977) in *Basic Prescriptions of Chinese Medicine of China*, 1988, p. 44.

34. Spirit of Ginseng, Antler and Tiger Bone

Ingredients:

Korean ginseng, rhizome bark of *Schizophragma integrifolium Oliv.* , eucommia bark (parched with salt), prepared Sichuan aconite root, myrrh (prepared), fleece-flower root (prepared), teasel root, nodular branch of pine, rhizome of polygonatum, root of cyathula, antler, prepared rhizome of rehmannice, earthworm, large-leaved gentian, loranthus mulberry mistletoe rhizome of Ligusticum Chuanxiong, cinnamom twig, Chinese wolfberry fruit, astragalus root, root of herbaceous peony (parched), mulberry twig, cane sugar, root of ledebouriella, wild aconite rhizome (prepared), Sichuan *Dioscorea hypolauca*, franincense, dried *Agkistrodon acutus*, root of Chinese climatis, safflower, glue of tiger bone, refined honey, spirit.

Actions:

Invigorates the spleen, replenishes *qi*, tonifies the blood to calm the mind, nourishes the liver and the kidney, warms *yang*, dispels cold and wind and promotes collateral flow.

Indications:

Paralysis (arthralgia including wandering and static pain, swelling pain in the extremities, deficiency of blood and *qi* and weak constitution), insomnia, dreaminess, lassitude of the extremities, pallor, palpitation, cold extremities, lack of appetite, pale tongue with white fur, soft, floating pulse, weakness of the waist and knees, numbness of the hands and feet, myophagism and pale tongue with white fur.

Cautions:

Do not take medicine containing pinellia, Trichosanthes kirilowi, hyacinth bletilla, ampelopsis and *Bulbus fritillariae* while taking the spirit and patients who have swelling arthralgia must not take it.

Source:

Medicinal Criteria of Zhejiang Province, (1978) in *Basic Prescriptions of Chinese Medicine of China*, vol. 1, 1988, p. 45.

35. *Fengliaoxing* Spirit

Ingredients:

Noterpterygium, root of Chinese climatis, rhizome of slender acanthopanax, *Erycibe obtusifolia*, cinnamom twig, rhizome of heracleum, seed of sweet wormwood, ephedra twig, root of Dahurian angelica, aniseed, Chinese angelica root, rhizome of Ligusticum Chuanxiong (prepared in spirit), capejasmine, spirits of 50% alcohol content, tetrandra root.

Actions:

Dispels wind and cold, activates collateral flow and alleviates pain.

Indications:

Paralysis due to wind-cold-dampness, numbness of the extremities, arthralgia and myalgia.

Cautions:

Patients who have *yin* deficiency or a fever due to cold must not take it.

Administration and Dosage:

Oral administration, 10—15ml doses, twice per day for

adults.

Source:

Medicinal Criteria of Anhui Province (1982) in *Basic Prescriptions of Chinese Medicine of China*, vol. 1, 1988, p. 61.

36. Spirit of Snakes

Ingredients:

fresh black-tail snake (without head and viscera), fresh *Bungarus multicinctus multicinctus* (without head and viscera), fresh cobra (without head and viscera), sargentgloryvine, *Climatis finetiana Levl. et Vant*, root of Chinese climatis ladybell root, hairy birthwort, *Parabarium micranthum Pier.*, vladimiria root, Chinese silkvine root bark, Chinese photinia, Sichuan aconite root, dried orange peel, rhizome of heracleum, achyranthes root, Chinese angelica root, sealwort, root of three-nerved spicebush, root of Dahurian angelica, *Celastrus orbiculatus*, rhizome of grass-leaved sweetflay, *Lycopodium clavatum L.*, loranthus mulberry mistletoe, wild aconite root, rhizome of Ligusticum Chuanxiong, cinnamom twig, Chinese cynomonium, licorice root, fruit of jujube, spirits.

Indications:

Arthralgia due to wind, cold and dampness. Its major symptoms are spasm, pain and numness of muscles and bones and joint rigidity; rheumatoid arthritis, rheumatic arthritis, sciatica brachial plexus neuritis, etc.

Administration and Dosage:

Oral administration, 15ml doses, twice per day. Children over 7 take half of the dose.

Cautions:

Pregnant women and those with decreased renal function must not take it.

Source:

Medicinal Criteria of Hunan Province, (1982) in *Basic Prescriptions of Chinese Medicine of China*, vol. 1, 1988, p. 61.

37. *Liufangteng* Spirit (highly toxic)

Ingredients:

Liufangteng rhizome, spirits *q. s.*

Pharmaceutical Process:

Dust the rhizome with a brush, cut or grind it into small pieces, let them soak in one half of the spirits in a sealed container for 3 days. Filtrate the infusion and let the herbs soak twice in spirits *q. s.* for 2 days each time. Filtrate the three infusions, mix the three filtrates and keep the mixture static for 3 days. Then filtrate it again and add spirits to increase its quantity to 1,000ml The medicated spirit is brown and clear liquid and each ml of it is equal to 0. 1 gram of the herbs in potency.

Actions:

Dispels wind and dampness.

Indication:

Rheumatic arthritis.

Administration and Dosage:

Oral administration, 5—15ml doses, 3 times per day. Children should take smaller doses in accordance with their condition.

Cautions:

It is highly toxic, so its dosage should be strictly restricted; do not eat cold or sour food, fish or bean products while taking it; pregnant women, nephropathic or debilitated patients must not take it; hypertension or heart patients should be cautious in taking it. Toxic reactions are nausea, vomiting, abdominal pain and inhibited breath and heartbeat. Steamed tea can be used as an antidote for minimal poisoning. Persons mildly poisoned can have enema and injections of cardiac stimulants like caffeine and coramine, etc. People seriously effected should have injections of cocculin or foxglove.

Source:

Pharmacopoeia of Rural Prescriptions of Chinese Herbal Medicine, ed. the Scientific and Technical Commission of Honghe Prefecture of Yunnan Province et al, 1976, p. 184.

38. *Shiguogong* Spirit

Ingredients:

Licorice 10 grams, noterpterygium 10 grams, rhizome of Ligusticum Chuanxiong, Chinese angelica root 15 grams, rhizome of heracleum 10 grams, teasel root 10 grams, silkworm excrement 15 grams, fruit of Chinese flowering quince 15 grams, achyranthes root 30 grams, ledebouriella root 20 grams, rhizome of polygonatum 50 grams, loranthus mulberry mistletoe 25 grams, rhizome of large-headed atractylodes 30 grams, safflower 15 grams, glue of antler 5 grams, glue of freshwater turtle shell, rice fermented with red yeast 60 grams.

Pharmaceutical Process:

Grind all the ingredients except the antler glue, the turtle shell glue and the rice and put them into a jar with the fermented rice. Add 18,000 grams of candy powder and 9,000 grams of spirits, heat the antler glue and turtle shell glue in spirits *q. s.*

respectively till the spirit boils, then pour them into the jar, seal it up and keep it static for at least 3 months. Filtrate them to obtain clear filtrate, press the dregs, keep the extract static and mix the filtrate with it. Then filtrate the mixture. It can also be made with the method of extraction by infusion in cold spirits.

Actions:

Dispels wind and dampness, nourishes the blood and activates the flow in the collaterals.

Indications:

Numbness of the limbs, arthralgia and arthralgia due to wind cold and dampness.

Caution:

Pregnant women should be cautious in taking it.

Administration and Dosage:

9—15 gram doses, 2 or 3 times per day while it is warm.

Source:

Pharmacopoeia of the People's Republic of China, Vol. 1, 1963, p. 350.

39. Spirit of Tiger Bone

Ingredients:

Prepared tiger bone, rhizome of Ligusticum Chuanxiong, Chinese angelica root, gastrodia tuber, rhizome or slender acanthopanax, safflower, teasel root, white eggplant root 30 grams each; fruit of Chinese flowering quince 90 grams, rhizome of polygonatum 60 grams, large-leaved gentian 15 grams, root of ledebouriella 15 grams, mulberry twig 120 grams.

Pharmaceutical Process:

Grind the ingredients together, put them with 10,000 grams

of spirits into a jar and seal it up. Stir them once per day for a week, then stir them once per week for four weeks. Filtrate them to obtain clear infusion, press the dregs and mix the extract with the clear infusion. Add 1,000 grams of melted rock candy, mix them well, keep the mixture static, and finally filtrate it.

Actions:

Dispels wind, cold and dampness to alleviate pain.

Indications:

Wind, cold and dampness that invade the channels and collaterals, stiffness and spasm of the muscles, numbness of the limbs, arthralgia, twisted eyes and month and severe and migratory arthralgia.

Administration and Dosage:

15—30 gram doses, twice per day while it is warm.

Caution:

Pregnant women must not take it.

Source:

Pharmacopoeia of the People's Republic of China, Vol. 1, 1963, p. 371. (The prescription is based on a recipe in *General Collection for Holy Relief* completed around 1111—1117).

40. Tiger Bone Spirit No. 1

Ingredients:

Tiger bone, seed of Job's tears, *Dioscorea hypoglauca*, *herba epimedii*, prepared rhizome of rehmannia, dried orange peel, rhizome of polygonatum and achyranthes root 240 grams each; Chinese angelica rhizome, rhizome of slender acanthopanax, green tangerine peel, root of herbaceous peony, prepared wild aconite rhizome, fruit of Chinese flowering quince, fruit of Chinese wolf berry, safflower, Asian *puccoon*, prepared Sichuan aconite rhizome, teasel root, noterpterygium root, root of Dahurian angelica, psoralea fruit, long-noded pit viper, eucommia bark, Tiantai lindera root, ledebouriella root, root, bark of tree peony, fingered citron, ginseng, amomum fruit, sandalwood, Chinese cassia bark, round cardamom, rhizome of birthwood, pilose antler cloves 15 grams each; nodular pine branch 120 grams, frankincense, and myrrh 60 grams each, musk 0. 6 gram, rice fermented with red yeast 375 grams; brown sugar 2,880 grams, honey 4,800 grams.

Pharmaceutical Process:

Decoct the tiger bone till it gets sticky, grind the ingredients from the seed of Job's tear to ginseng together, grind the ingredients from the amomum fruit to pilose antler into small pieces, grind the frankincense and myrrh into fine powder and sift it. Then grind it with the musk into fine powder, sift the powder, and put 33,000 grams of spirits, the rice fermented with red yeast, brown sugar and honey into a jar. Add the prepared ingredients mentioned above, cover the jar, put it into a larger container with water and heat it till the spirit boils. Pour the decoction into a container, seal it up, keep it static for at least 3 months, then filtrate it to obtain clear liquid. Press the dregs, keep the extract static, mix it with the clear filtrate and finally filtrate it or percolate it.

Actions:

Dispels wind and dampness.

Indications:

Arthralgia due to wind, cold and dampness, numbness of the hands and feet, myalgia and soreness and weakness of the waist.

Administration and Dosage:

15 gram doses, twice per day while it is warm.

Cautions:

Pregnant women and people with deficinecy of *yin* and hyperactivity of internal fire must not take it.

Source:

Pharmacopoeia of the People's Republic of China, Vol. 1, 1963, p. 371.

41. Tiger Bone Spirit No. 2

Ingredients:

Tiger tibia (infused in spirit and crisp fried in a liquid), *Dioscorea hypoglauca*, achyranthes root (soaked in spirit for a night), *Fpimedium brevicornum F. koreanum*, seed of Job's tears, prepared rhizome of rehmannia (sprinkled with spirit, steamed and dried in sunlight 9 times) 60 grams each.

Pharmaceutical Process:

Grind them into small pieces, put them into a silk bag and let them soak in spirit.

Actions:

Dispels wind, nourishes the blood, replenishes *qi* and strengthens the muscles and bones.

Indications:

Numbness and pain in the feet, knees, waist and legs.

Dosage:

10ml each time.

Source:

Effective Prescriptions for Universal Relief, Vol. 4

42. Tiger Bone Spirit No. 3

Ingredients:

Tiger tibia (crisp fried in a liquid) 105 grams, Chinese angelica root (washed in spirits and baked), prepared aconite root (stir-baked and barked), Sichuan aconite root (stir-baked and barked) 45 grams each; noterpterygium root, rhizome of Ligusticum Chuanxiong, rhizome of heracleum, root of herbaceous peony, eucommia bark (without the outermost covering and parched with ginger), *Dioscorea hypoglauca*, ledebouriella root, cassia bark (without the outermost covering), desertliving cistanche (washed in spirit), rhizome of cythula (washed in spirit), astragalus root, *Cibotium barometz J. Sm.* (with the villus burnt up), *Poria cocos*, tribulus fruit (parched to remove the thorns), ginseng, gastrodia tuber, teasel root 30 grams.

Pharmaceutical Process:

Grind them into small pieces, put them into a silk bag, soak them in limeless wine and seal up the bottle for 3 days in spring, 2 days in summer, 7 days in autumn or 10 days in winter.

Indications:

Arthralgia due to wind, carpopedal pains, difficulty in walking and weakness of the legs and knees.

Administration and Dosage:

1 cup each time before meal. Bake the dregs, make them into pills with spirits and take them with warm spirits.

Source:

Effective Formulas Handed Down for Generations, *Vol.* 13

43. Tiger Bone Spirit No. 4

Ingredients:

Tiger bone (fried in a liquid to obtain yellow juice and

pounded into pieces as small as a sparrow's head); rice 3 *dan* (= 3 hectolitres) and distiller's yeast 4 *dou* (=4 decalitres).

Pharmaceutical Process:

Add 3 *dan* of water, brew them in a normal way and keep them airtight for 50 days.

Indications:

Arthralgia and myalgia.

Source:

Prescriptions for Emergencies, *Vol.* 19

44. Tiger Bone Spirit No. 5

Ingredients:

Tiger bone crisp fried in a liquid 10 grams, Mongolian gazelle horn 30 grams, root of herbaceous peony 60 grams.

Phamarceutical Process:

Let the ingredients soak in spirits airtight for 7 days, shaking the container frequently (14 days in autumn or winter).

Actions:

Nourishes the kidney, consolidates the bones and dispels wind to relieve pain.

Indications:

Deficiency of the kidney-*qi*, arthralgia of the limbs due to the invasion of pathogenic wind into the channels, collaterals, muscles, tendons and bones.

Administration and Dosage:

10ml before meal per day.

Storage:

Keep it airtight in a dark and cool place.

Source:

A Dictionary of Chinese Medicine.

45. Tiger Bone Spirit No. 6

Ingredients:

Tiger bone (crisp fried in a liquid).

Pharmaceutical Process:

Pound it into small pieces and brew spirit with them.

Indications:

Arthralgia due to wind, cold and dampness.

Source:

Fssentials Of Diet, Vol. *Spirits*

46. Spirit of *Erycibe Obtusifolia*

Ingredients:

Erycibe obtusifolia 1,000 grams, cinnamom twig 30 grams, ephedra twig 37.5 grams, noterpterygium 3 grams, Chinese angelica root 3 grams, rhizome of Ligusticum Chuanxiong 3 grams, root of Dahurian angelica 3 grams, psoralea fruit 3 grams, frankincense 3 grams, *Gleditsia sinensis* 3 grams, dried orange peel 13 grams, rhizome of Chinese atractylodes 3 grams, bark of official magnolia 3 grams, nutgrass flatsedge rhizome 3 grams, aucklandia root 3 grams, fruit of *Poncirus trifoliata* 20 grams rhizome of large-headed atractylodes, Chinese yam 3 grams, Siberian solomonseal rhizome 8 grams, dodder seed 3 grams, aniseed 3 grams, bitter almonds 3 grams, rhizome of oriental water plantain 3 grams, trogopterus dung 3 grams, silkworm excrement 6.5 grams.

Pharmaceutical Process:

Steam the *Erycibe obtusifolia* for 2 hours, put it into a container with the other ingredients, add 4,250ml. of spirits and seal it up. Let them soak in the spirit for 40 days, heating it 2 3 times to 35 degrees centigrade. Finally, filtrate the infusion.

Actions:

Dispels wind and dampness, dissipates blood stasis to stop pain.

Indications:

Arthralgia due to wind, cold and dampness, numbness of the hands and feet, soreness and pains in the waist and legs and traumatic injury.

Administration and Dosage:

Oral administration, 1—15 ml. doses, 2—3 times per day. An affected part can be topically treated and if it is sore, painful and black, add the spirit to pounded and parched ginger and smear on the part.

Caution:

Pregnant women must not take it, but can use it externally except on the abdomen.

Source:

Pharmacopoeia of the People's Republic of China, Vol. 1, 1977, p. 678.

47. Spirit of Wasps

Ingredient:

Wasps 100 grams.

Pharmaceutical Process:

Let the wasps soak in 1,000ml of spirit for 15 days and filtrate them.

Actions:

Dispels wind and dampness.

Administration and Dosage:

Oral administration, 15—25ml doses, twice per day.

48. Spirit of Flowering Quince

Ingredients:

Fruit of Chinese flowering quince 45 grams, loranthus mulberry mistletoe 75 grams, rhizome of polygonatum 240 grams, teasel root 30 grams, rhizome of cyathula 90 grams, Chinese angelica root 45 grams, rhizome of Ligusticum Chuanxiong 60 grams, safflower 45 grams, rhizome of heracleum 80 grams, noterpterygium 30 grams, ledebouriella root 60 grams, rhizome of large—headed atractylodes 90 grams, silkworm excrement 60 grams, rice fermented with red yeast 180 grams, licorice root 30 grams.

Pharmaceutical Process:

Grind all the ingredients except the rice to small pieces, dissolve 555 grams of brown sugar in 1, 100 grams of spirits and percolate them. Using the mixture of sugar and spirit as solution, let them soak for 48 hours, then percolate them at a speed of 1—3ml per minute. Keep the percolate static and filtrate it.

Actions:

Dispels wind and dampness, relaxes the muscles and tendons and activates the flow of *qi* and blood in the channels and collaterals.

Indications:

Arthralgia due to wind, cold and dampness and numbness of the limbs.

Administration and Dosage:

Oral administration, twice per day and 20—30ml each time.

Caution:

Pregnant women should be cautious in taking it.

Source:

Pharmacopoeia of the People's Republic of China, Vol. 1, 1977, p. 839.

49. Rheumatism Spirit

Ingredients:

Chinese angelica 120 grams, spatholobus stem 180 grams, root of herbaceous peony 150 grams, prepared Sichuan aconite root 60 grams, prepared rhizome of rehmannia 180 grams, large-leaved gentian 120 grams, *Herba Epimedii* 90 grams, licorice, root 60 grams, loranthus mulberry mistletoe 120 grams, astragalus root 180 grams, earthworm 90 grams, safflower 60 grams, sugar 500 grams, spirit 5,000ml.

Pharmaceutical Process:

Cut the ingredients into slices or grind them into small pieces, wet them with spirits *q. s.*, put them into an extractor and add spirits q. s. Heat them, extract them for 2 hours, get the medicated spirit and add spirits q. s. Heat them and extract them again for 2 hours, mix the extracts, put the mixture into an enamel cup, add spirit q. s. and seal it up. Let the mixture soak in the spirit for 3 weeks, filtrate it to obtain clear extract, press the dregs, filtrate them, mix the extract with the extract mentioned before and add a certain amount of sugar. Keep the mixture static to dissolve the sugar, filtrate it and pack it separately.

Actions:

Dispels wind and dampness, removes the obstruction in the channels and collaterals and promotes blood circulation to alleviate pain.

Indications:

Rheumatic arthritis, lumbago and numbness of the hands and feet, etc.

Administration and Dosage:

Oral administration, 5ml doses, three times per day.

Source:

Institute of Chinese Medicine and Medicinal Herbs of Shanxi Province, *Pharmaceutical Techniques of Chinese Medicine*, 1982, p. 214.

50. Spirit of Slender Acanthopanax

Ingredients:

Chinese angelica 120 grams, orientavine 120 grams, futokadsura stem 120 grams, rhizome of Ligusticum Chuanxiong 120 grams, root of Chinese climatis 120 grams, rhizome of large-headed atractylodes 180 grams, root of Dahurian angelica 180 grams, achyranthes root 240 grams, safflower 240 grams, rhizome of slender acanthopanax 500 grams, root of *codonopsis pilosula* 720 grams, rhizome of common turmeric 720 grams, rhizome of heracleum 60 grams, prepared Sichuan aconite root 60 grams, prepared wild aconite root 60 grams, rhizome of polygonatum 1, 920 grams, nutmeg (roasted in talcum powder) 90 grams, sandalwood 120 grams, chrysanthemum flower 240 grams, seed of Amomum kravanh 90 grams, buds of *Syzygium aromaticum Merr. et Perry* 60 grams, amomum fruit 60 grams, capejasmine 1,500 grams, dried orange peel 500 grams, cassia bark 60 grams, aucklandia root 60 grams, rock candy 19,200 grams, spirits 192,000 grams.

Pharmaceutical Process:

Cut the herbs from the angelica root to the rhizome of polygonatum into slices or grind them, then grind the ingredients from the nutmeg to the candy. Put the first seventeen ingredients into a copper pot, submerge them with clear water and decoct them, adding water when necessary. Obtain extract once every 2—4 hours. Add clear water to the dregs, decoct them, and repeat the step 3—4 times. Then press the dregs, remove them and mix the extracts. Keep the mixture static, filtrate it, then heat it, reducing the fire as the medicinal liquid gets increasingly thick and stirring it with a bronze laddle or a stick to prevent it from burning. When it is thick enough, put a few drops on a piece of blotting paper to see if they are absorbed in order to test their thickness. Pour the spirit into a stainless steel pot, add the thick medicinal liquid and the remaining ingredients and put the pot into a boiling cauldron to heat them till the spirit boils. 6—8 minutes later, take out the pot, pour the medicine into a jug, seal it up and let the ingredients soak in the spirit for 3—5 months. Filtrate them to obtain clear liquid, press the dregs, filtrate them, mix the extract with the clear liquid, keep the mixture static for some time and pack it.

Actions:

Dispels dampness and wind, relaxes the muscles and tendons and promotes the flow of *qi* and blood in the channels and collaterals.

Indications:

Stiffness and spasm of the hands and feet due to wind and cold, numbness of the limbs, a sensation of soreness and heaviness in the waist and knees, damp renal capsules and coldness of the female genitals.

Administration and Dosage:

Oral administration, 15—30ml doses, 3 times per day while it is warm.

Storage:

Keep it airtight in a dark and cool place.

Source:

Institute of Chinese Medicine and Medicinal Herbs of Shanxi Province, *Pharmaceutical Techniques of Chinese Medicine*, 1982, p. 216.

51. Spirit of Seed of Job's Tears

Ingredients:

Seed of Job's tears and achyranthes root 60 grams each; bark of tobira, rhizome of slender acanthopanax, parched fruit of *Ponicirus trifoliata*, rhizome of heracleum, ledebouriella root, eucommia bark (crisp fried with ginger juice) 30 grams each; rhizome of large—headed atractylodes 15 grams; dried glutinous rehmannia 45 grams.

Pharmaceutical Process:

Grind the ingredients into small pieces, put them into a silk bag and let them soak in 5 litres of good spirit for 14 days. Soak them in spirits separately in summer.

Indication:

Podalic arthralgia.

Administration and Dosage:

3—4 times per day and 10—15 ml each time before meals while it is warm.

Source:

A Classified Book on Treating Exogenous Fabrile Disease,
Vol. 18

52. Spirit of Astragalus

Ingredients:

Astragalus root, ledebouriella root, root of *Asarum heterotropodies mandshuricum*, rhizome of Ligusticum Chuanxiong and achyranthes root 45 grams each; prepared aconite root, Sichuan pepper, stir—fried licorice root 30 grams each; Sichuan aconite root, dogwood fruit, large—headed gentian and pueraria root 21 grams each.

Pharmaceutical Process:

Soak the herbs in spirit.

Indications:

Arthralgia and numbness.

Administration and Dosage:

3 times per day.

Remarks:

Add desertliving cistanche to treat deficiency syndrome, stem of *Clematic apiifolia DC*. to treat diarrhea and steam of noble dendrobium and calamus to treat amnesia.

Source:

A Dictionary of Chinese Medicine

53. Spirit of Slender Acanthopanax

Ingredients:

Rhizome of slender acanthopanax, parched thorns of *Poncirus trifoliata*, root bark of *zhujiao*, red sage root and seed of Job's tears 240 grams each; rhizome of Ligusticum Chuanxiong, stir-baked ginger 150 grams each; root bark of shaggy fruited dittany, large-leaved gentian, akebi, stir-baked thin and long root of wild aconite and licorice root stir-fried in a liquid 120 grams each; hemp seed 3 *sheng* (=3 litres), dried bark of Cinnamomum cassia (without the outermost covering) and Chinese angelica root 90 grams each.

Pharmaceutical Process:

Grind the herbs into small pieces, put them into a silk bag and let them soak in 3 decalitres of spirit for 3—4 days in spring or summer or for 6—7 days in autumn or winter.

Indications:

Arthralgia, mental depression, pale face, stiffness and spasm of the muscles and tendons, difficulty in stretching the limbs and abdominal spasms.

Administration and Dosage:

0. 2—0. 3 litre doses at first and increased the dosage later. Take it while warm.

Source:

Miraculous Cures, Vol, 38

54. Spirit of Snakes

Ingredients:

Black-tail snake, pallas-pit viper, cobra.

Indications:

Rheumatoid arthritis and rheumatoid spinal osteoarthritis.

Administration and Dosage:

25—50ml doses once or twice per day.

Source:

Plantation of Medicinal Experiment of Hangzhou, Zhejiang

Province, *Selection of the Materials of the National Exhibition of chinese Medicinal Herbs and New Therapy*, 1972, p. 205.

55. Spirit of *Kniphofia Uvaria*

Ingredients:

root of *kniphofia uvaria* 100 grams, spirits 1,000ml.

Pharmaceutical Process:

Cut the root into small pieces, put them into a container, add one half of the spirits and seal up the container. Let the root pieces soak in the spirits for 7 days, then pour out the clear part of it, add the remaining spirit and seal up the container. Let the root pieces soak for 4 days, pour out the clear part of the infusion and mix the two clear infusions. Keep the mixture static for 3 days and filtrate it. It contains about 45% alcohol.

Actions:

Dispels wind and dampness.

Indication:

Rheumatoid arthritis.

Administration and Dosage:

Oral administration, 10—20ml. dose, 3 times per day. Children should take smaller doses according to their condition.

Source:

Norms of Rural Preparations of Chinese Medicinal Herbs of Yunnan Province, Vol. 1, 1977, p. 53.

56. Spirit of Delavay Ampelopsis

Ingredients:

Toddalia asiatica Lam. 50 grams, *Periploca forrestii Schltr.* 50 grams, root of Delavay ampelopsis 50 grams, *Chloranthus henryi Hemsl* 50 grams, giant knotweed rhizome 50 grams, eucommia

98

bark 50 grams, sargentgloryvine 50 grams, rhizome of *Wisteria Venusta Rehd. et wils* 50 grams, *Kadsura oblongifolia Merr.* 50 grams, 50% proof spirit 5,000ml.

Pharmaceutical Process:

Wash the herbs clean, cut them into slices and dry them. Let them soak in the spirits for 2 weeks, stirring them once a day in the first week, then filtrate them and mix the two filtrates of about 4,000ml in all.

Actions:

Promotes the flow of *qi* and blood in the channels and collaterals and dispels cold and dampness.

Indications:

Rheumatic arthritis.

Administration and Dosage:

Oral administration, 10—20ml doses, twice per day in the morning and the evening.

Source:

Norms of Rural Preparations of Chinese Medicinal Herbs of Yunnan Province, Vol. 1, 1977, p. 53.

57. Rheumatic Arthritis Spirit

Ingredients:

Rogersflower rhizome, climbing entada stem, stem of *Kadsura longipedunculata Finet* 17 grams each; *Speranskia tuberculata Baill.* 13 grams, *Pedilanthus tithymaloides Poit* 3 grams, jujube fruit 35 grams.

Pharmaceutical Process:

Pound the ingredients into small pieces, let them infuse in 1,000ml of spirit for 10 days. Filtrate them, let the dregs infuse in 500ml of spirit for 5 days, filtrate them, mix the two filtrates well and pack the mixture into a bottle.

Actions:

Dispels wind and dampness, relaxes the muscles and tendons and promotes the flow of *qi* and blood in the channels and collaterals.

Indications:

Traumatic injury and rheumatic arthritis.

Administration and Dosage:

Oral administration, 10—15ml doses twice per day (can also be applied topically to the affected part).

Source:

Norms of Rural Preparations of Chinese Medicinal Herbs of Yunnan Province, Vol. 1, 1977, p. 54

58. Spirit of Dog Bone Glue

Ingredients:

Dog bone glue 100 grams, *Dioscorea nipponica Mak.* 150 grams, southern wine 330 ml., 65% alcohol content spirit *q. s.*

Pharmaceutical Process:

Grind the *Dioscorea nipponica Mak.* into small pieces, let them soak in some of the spirit for 72 hours before percolating them to obtain 600ml of percolate. Dissolve the glue in the wine, mix it with the percolate and add the remaining spirits to increase its quantity to 1,000ml. Mix them well, keep the mixture static at room temperature, then filtrate it and pack it.

Actions:

Dispels cold to relieve pain, removes wind, promotes the flow of blood and strengthens the muscles, tendons and bones.

Indications:

Rheumatic arthritis, etc.

Administration and Dosage:

20—30ml doses, 3 times per day.

Source:

Chinese Medicinal Herbs, Issue 5, 1977. p. 21.

59. Preparation of Dog Bone Glue

Ingredients:

Dog bones 1, 000 grams, rock candy 14 grams, bean oil 3 grams, southern wine 2 grams.

Process:

Pound the bones into strips 3—5 *cun* long, let them soak in water for 2—3 days and decoct them till the decoction gets thick, repeating the step several times. Mix the decoctions, add a little alum, keep the mixture static, then concentrate its clear part. Add the candy, oil and wine, mix them well, then put the mixture into a glue—congealing box and slice it or dice it when it congeals.

Source:

Ibid.

60. Spirit of Panther Bone

Ingredients:

Panther bone 80 grams, *Epimedium brevicomum E. koreanum* (prepared with sheep oil), rhizome of polygonatum, seed of Job's tears, *Dioscorea hypoglauca*, dried orange peel, achyranthes root 80 grams each; Chinese angelica root, rhizome of slender acan-thopanax, root of herbaceous peony, prepared Sichuan aconite root, safflower, lithosperm root, noterpterygium root, root of Dahurian angelica, green tangerine peel, rhizome of Ligusticum

Chuanxiong, psoralea fruit (prepared with salt), eucommia bark, Agkistrodon acutus (without head), amomum fruit, cassia bark (without outermost covering), round cardamon (shelled), ledebouriella root, finger citron fruit, peony bark, ginseng, rhizome of birthwood, cloves, pilose antler 5 grams each; nodular branch of pine 40 grams, musk 0.2 gram, frankincense and myrrh 20 grams each; rice fermented with red yeast 200 grams, brown sugar 960 grams, honey 1, 600 grams, spirit 17,600 ml.

Pharmaceutical Process:

Decoct the panther bone till all of its glue is extracted, filtrate the decoction and concentrate the filtrate. Grind the frankincense, musk and myrrh into fine pieces and grind all the remaining ingredients into small pieces except the rice, sugar, honey and spirit. Put all the ingredients into a percolator, percolate them, press the dregs, filtrate them, mix the filtrate with the percolate and pack the mixture separately.

Actions:

Dispels wind and dampness.

Indications:

Arthralgia due to wind, cold and dampness, numbness of the feet and hands, and weakness of the waist and knees.

Administration and Dosage:

Oral administration, 15ml doses, twice per day.

Cautions:

Pregnant women and patients who have deficiency of *yin* and hyperactivity of internal fire must not take it.

Source:

Medicinal Criteria of Henan Province, 1977

61. Spirit of Rehmannia

Ingredients:

Rhizome of rehmannia 480 grams, soy beans (prepared) and poplar bark 240 grams each, ginger (minced and stir-fried in a liquid) 60 grams.

Pharmaceufical Process:

Put the ingredients into a silk bag , put the bag into a china jug and let them soak airtight in spirit for 7 days.

Indications:

Pains in the waist and feet.

Administration and Dosage:

10ml before meals while it is hot.

Source:

Peaceful Holy Benevolent Prescriptions, *Vol.* 44

62. Spirit of Chinese Angelica

Ingredients:

Safflower 55 grams, Chinese angelica root 80 grams, prepared aconite root 55 grams, *Schisandra propiqua Baill. var. sinensis Oliv* 80 grams, spirits 1, 000 grams.

Pharmaceutical Process:

Cut the herbs into slices and let them soak in the spirit for 10 days.

Actions:

Promotes blood circulation and dissipates blood stasis to relieve pain.

Indication:

Pain induced by hyperosteogeny.

Administration and Dosage:

Oral administration, 10—20ml doses (no more than 20ml), twice per day in the morning and evening.

Source:

Rural Preparations of Chinese Medicinal Herbs of Guizhou, 1977, p. 202.

63. Spirit of Snakes

Ingredients:

Black-tail snake 1,500 grams, *Agkistrodon acutus* 200 grams, *Ophisaurus harti Boulenger* 100 grams, rhizome of Chinese foxglove 500 grams, rock candy 5,000 grams spirits 100,000 grams.

Pharmaceufical Process:

Cut off the heads of the snakes, wash them in spirits and dry them; wash the foxglove root clean and mince it. Put the candy into a pot, add water, heat it till the candy melts and turns yellow, then filtrate it with gauze. Now pour the spirit into a jar, add the snakes and herbs, seal up the jar, and stir the infusion once per day for 10—15 days. Filtrate it, add the candy, mix them well and filtrate the mixture.

Actions:

Dispels wind and cold, removes the obstruction in the channels and collaterals, dissipates bloods stasis, relieves convulsion, removes pathogenic heat and nourishes *yin* and the tendons.

Indications:

Arthralgia and myalgia due to wind, cold and dampness, numbness of the limbs, difficulty in stretching them, hemiparalysis, blood stasis induced by traumatic injury, convulsion due to the invasion of pathogenic wind into the collaterals, bone tuberculosis and sequela of shock.

Source:

Chinese Medicated Dietetics of Tongrentang of Chengdu, 1985, p. 184.

64. Wine of Chinese Angelica

Ingredients:

Chinese angelica 60 grams, millet wine 1, 000 grams.

Pharmaceutical Process:

Cut the herb into slices, and let them soak in the wine for 7 days.

Indication:

Lingering and fixed pains in the arms.

Administration and Dosage:

10—20ml doese, twice per day.

Source:

Chinese Medicated Dietetics, 1985, p. 202.

65. Spirit of Gastrodia

Ingredients:

Gastrodia tuber 30 grams, spirits 500 grams.

Pharmaeutical Process:

Let the herb soak in the spirit for 7 days.

Indications:

Arthralgia due to wind dampness and numbness of the limbs.

Administration and Dosage:

10—20ml doses, 2—3 times per day.

Source:

Chinese Medicated Dietetics, 1985, p. 248.

66. Spirit of Cibot

Ingredients:

Cibot rhizome slices 20 grams, *Cinnamomum camphora Presl* and European *vebean* 12 grams each; eucommia bark and teasel root 15 grams each; root of Chinese climatis 10 grams, red achyranthes root 6 grams, spirits 1,000 grams.

Pharmaceutical Process:

Let the herbs soak in the spirit for 7 days.

Indications:

Myalgia due to wind and dampness and weakness of the waist and knees.

Administration and Dosage:

20—30ml doses, twice per day.

Source:

Chinese Medicated Dietetics, 1985, p. 227.

67. Spirit of Roses

Ingredients:

Roses (without stamens, pistils and bases and dried in a dark place), safflower, Chinese angelica 10 grams each.

Pharmaceutical Process:

Decoct them, remove the dregs and mix the extract with good spirits.

Indication:

Arthralgia due to wind.

Administration and Dosage:

7 doses.

Source:

Mirror of Medicinal Herbs

68. Spirit of Loofah

Ingredients:

Loofah 150 grams, spirits 500ml.

Pharmaceufical Process:

Let the loofah soak in the spirit for 7 days and remove the dregs.

Indication:

Arthralgia.

Administration and Dosage:

10ml each time.

Source:

Chinese Dietetic Therapy, p. 374

69. Spirit of Plum

Ingredients:

Plum, spirits *q. s.*

Pharmaceutical Process:

Let the plum soak in spirits 2cm above it for a month.

Indication:

Arthralgia due to wind and dampness.

Administration and Dosage:

Take it separately or apply it to the affected part.

Source:

Chinese Dietetic Therapy, *p.* 374.

70. Spirit of Pepper

Ingredients:

Pepper 12 grams, spirits 500 grams.

Pharmaceutical Process:

Let the peppers soak in the spirit for half a month.

Indications:

Rheumatic arthritis, etc.

Administration and Dosage:

15ml doses, twice per day.

Source:

Chinese Dietetic Therapy, p. 374

71. Spirit of Glossy Pivet

Ingredients:

Bark of glossy pivet.

Pharmaceutical Process:

Wash the bark clean, cut it into slices, let them soak in the spirit and decoct them.

Indications:

Rheumatic arthritis and weakness of the waist and knees.

Administration and Dosage:

Oral administration.

Source:

A Handbook of Family Dietetic Therapy, 1982, p. 511.

72. Spirit of Seed of Job's Tears

Ingredient:

Ground seed of Job's tears *q. s.*

Pharmaceutical Process:

Brew the powder with distiller's yeast and rice or put it into a bag and decoct it in spirits.

Actions:

Dispels wind and dampness and strengthens the tendons, bones, spleen and stomach.

Administration and Dosage:

108

Oral administration.

Source:

A Handbook of Family Dietetic Therapy, 1982, p. 511.

73. Spirit of White Quartz

Ingredients:

White quartz and magnetite (calcined) 150 grams each.

Pharmaceutical Process:

Calcine and temper the quartz and magetite 7 times, put them into a silk bag and let them soak in 1. 000 ml of spirits for 5 —6 days.

Indications:

Arthralgia due to wind and dampness, deficiency of the kidney and deafness.

Administration and Dosage:

Oral administration while it is warm.

Source:

A Handbook of Family Dietetic Therapy, 1982, p. 511.

74. Spirit of Ursine Seal

Ingredients:

Ursine seal's penis and testes.

Pharmaceutical Process:

Cut them open, stir-fry them in a liquid to make them crisp, then grind them into powder and decoct 3—6 grams in spirits per dose.

Indication:

Heel pain.

Administration:

Oral administration while it is warm.

Source:

Chinese Dietetic Therapy, p. 306.

75. Spirit of Safflower

Ingredients:

Safflower 30 grams, spirits 500 grams.

Pharmaceutical Process:

Let it soak in the spirits for 7 days.

Benefits:

Promotes blood circulation, removes obstruction in the collateral and channels and subdues swelling to relieve pain.

Indication:

Pains due to blood stasis.

Administration and Dosage:

20—30ml doses, 2—3 times per day.

Source:

Chinese Medicated Dietetics, 1985, p. 262.

76. Spirit of Aconite Root and Seed of Job's Tears

Ingredients:

Prepared aconite root 180 grams, seed of Job's tears 120 grams, spirits 1,000 grams.

Pharmaceutical Process:

Let the herbs soak in the spirits for 15 days.

Indications:

Deficiency of blood, rheumatic lumbago, numbness of the limbs and dizziness.

Administration and Dosage:

Twice per day and 15 ml. each time.

Source:

77. Spirit of Flowering Quince

Ingredients:

Fruit of Chinese flowering quince 100 grams, loranthus mulberry mistletoe 50 grams, *Epimedium brevicornum E. koreanum* 50 grams, spirits 1,500 ml.

Pharmaceutical Process:

Let the herbs soak in the spirits for 7—10 days.

Indication:

Arthralgia.

Administration and Dosage:

20—30ml doses, once per day in the evening.

Source:

1,100 *Folk Prescriptions of Dietetic Therapy*, 1992, p. 124.

78. Spirit of Slender Acanthopanax

Ingredients:

rhizome of slender acathopanax 30 grams, fruit of Chinese wolfberry 30 grams, eucommia bark 30 grams, spirits 1,500ml.

Pharmaceutical Process:

Let the herbs soak in the spirits for 1 week.

Indication:

Arthralgia.

Administration and Dosage:

30ml doses, once per day before sleep.

Source:

1, 100 *Folk Prescriptions of Dietetic Therapy*, 1992, p. 125.

79. Spirit of Giant Knotweed and *Codonopsis Pilosula*

Ingredients:

Root of *Codonopsis pilosual* 100 grams, giant knotweed 100 grams, spirits 1, 500 grams.

Pharmaceutical Process:

Wash the herbs clean, drip-dry them, and let them soak in the spirits for 7 days.

Indication:

Arthralgia.

Administration and Dosage:

30 gram doses, once per day before sleep.

Source:

1, 100 *Folk Prscriptions of Dietetic Therapy*, 1992, p. 127.

80. Arthralgia Spirit

Ingredients:

Ginseng 10 grams, antler glue (melted by heating) and fruit of Chinese flowering quince 60 grams each; rock candy 250 grams, spirits 1, 500 grams.

Pharmaceutical Process:

Cut the ginseng and the quince fruit into thin slices and let them and the glue soak in the spirits for a month.

Actions:

Relieves arthralgia and myalgia due to wind and builds up health.

Indications:

Senile deficiency of *qi* and blood and arthralgia and myalgia.

Administration and Dosage:

10ml. before sleep.

Source:

Therapeutic and Invigorative Uses of Tonic Medicine, 1984,

p. 12.

81. Spirit of Chinese Holly Leaves

Ingredients:

Chinese holly leaves 100 grams, spirit 1, 000 grams.

Pharmaceutical Process:

Let the leaves infuse in the spirit for 10 days.

Actions:

Nourishes the liver and the kidneys and cures arthralgia.

Administration and Dosage:

10ml. before sleep.

Source:

Pharmaceutical Annals of Hunan

82. Spirit of Chinese Flowering Quince

Ingredients:

Noterpterygium root, rhizome of heracleum, fruit of Chinese flowering quince, bark of eucommia (parched), mulberry twig, white eggplant root, safflower, rhizome of slender acanthopanax, rhizome of rehmannia, prepared rhizome of rehmannia and rhizome of polygonatum 90 grams each, root of ledebouriella, root bark of *Schizophragma intergrifolium Oliv.*, prepared aconite root (soaked to remove the bark), rhizome of Ligusticum Chuanxiong, root of *Codonopsis pilosula*, white chrysanthemum flower, root of spikenard, cinnamon twig, root of Dahurian angelica, astragalus root (stir-fried in a liquid), licorice root, root of herbaceous peony (parched), gastrodia tuber, loranthus mulberry mistletoe, rhizome of *Homelomena occulata*, fruit of Chinese wolfberry, dried orange peel and rubia root 60 grams each, seed of round cardamon, pseudo-ginseng, fruit of amomum, aniseed, Chinese angelica root, deboned snake, and rice fermented with red yeast 30 grams each; tiger bone glue 120 grams, fruit of jujube 240 grams, rock candy 20, 000 grams.

Pharmaceutical Process:

Make wine from them.

Actions:

Dispels wind and cold, warms the channels and collaterals and promotes the flow of *qi* and blood in them and relaxes the muscles and tendons to alleviate pain.

Indications:

Arthralgia due to wind, cold and dampness, numbness of the limbs and traumatic injury.

Administration and Dosage:

Oral administration, 10—15ml doses, twice per day.

Caution:

Do not take more than the prescribed dose to prevent intoxication

Source:

Practical Preparations of Chinese Medicine in *Pharmacopoeia of Preparations of Chinese Medicine*, 1991, p. 258.

83. Arthralgia Spirit

Ingredients:

Spirits 8, 000 grams, sugar 800 grams, Chinese angelica root, ledebouriella root and ephedra twig 30 grams each; large-leaved gentian, psoradea fruit (prepared with salt), rhizome of heracleum, teasel root, safflower, noterpterygium root, gastrodia tuber, rhizome of Ligusticum Chuanxiong, resinous excretion from the fruit of Daemonorops draco and related *spp* (Palmae), frankincense, myrrh and rice fermented with red yeast 20 grams each; achyranthes root, fruit of Chinese flowering quince, *Artemisia anomala*, eucommia bark (prepared with salt), ground beetle, wild aconite root and root of Dahurian angelica 10 grams each; lithosperm root 8 grams.

Pharmaceutical Process:

Make wine from them.

Actions:

Dispels wind and cold, relaxes the muscles and tendons and promotes the flow of *qi* and blood in the channels and collaterals.

Indications:

Arthralgia due to wind, cold and dampness, traumatic injury (with symptoms of wandering or static arthralgia which worsens when it is cold and lessens when it is warm).

Administration and Dosage:

Oral administration, 10—15ml doses, twice per day.

Cautions:

Do not take it with rhinoceros horn, fritillary bulb, fruit—rind of Chinese trichosanthes, tuber of pinellia, bletilla tuber and ampelopsis root; do not take more than the prescriped dose.

84. *Guogong* Spirit

Ingredients:

Spirits, brown sugar, honey, rhizome of polygonatum, dried orange peel, rice fermented with red yeast, cassia bark, cloves, amomum fruit, round cardamom, rhizome of birthwood, sandalwood and Guogong extract from the infusion of spirits, rhizome of rehmannia, herb of common heron's bill, Chinese angelica root, achyranthes root, fruit of *Ponicirus trifoliata*, dried orange

peel, tuber of dwarf lilyturf, rhizome of large-headed atractylodes, rhizome of Chinese atractylodes, betel nut, rhizome of
Ligusticum Chuanxiong, fruit of Chinese flowering quince, root
of Dahurian angelica, peony root bark, noterpterygium root, magnolia bark, wrinkled giant hyssop, safflower, rhizome of heracleum, fruit of Chinese wolfberry, root of herbaceous peony, psoralea fruit, fingered citron, haw, capejasmine, Chinese wildvine
root bark, lithosperm root and ledebouriella root, etc.

Pharmaceutical Process:

Make wine from them.

Actions:

Dispels wind and dampness, promotes blood circulation, removes the obstruction in the channels and collaterals, replenishes
the liver and the kidney and strengthens the tendons and bones.

Indications:

Arthralgia due to wind, cold and dampness, rheumatic lumbago and numbness of the limbs.

Administration and Dosage:

Oral administration, 10—15ml doses, twice per day.

Cautions:

Pregnant women must not take it and do not take more than
the prescribed dose to prevent intoxication.

Source:

Practical Preparations of Chinese Medicine in *Preparations
of Chinese Medicine*, 1991, p. 253.

85. Spirit of *Akgistrodon Acutus*

Ingredients:

Akgistrodon acutus (wash it clean in warm water, cut 3 *cun* off its head and tail, soak it in spirit and bone it) 30 grams; scorpion 6 grams; Chinese angelica root, ledebouriella root, noterpterygium root, root of Dahurian angelica, gastrodia root, red peony root bark, licorice root, spatholobus stem, chrysanthemum flower and fruit of Chinese flowering quince 15 grams each; nux-vomica seed (stir-fried in a liquid) 9 grams; frankincense, myrrh, *Erodium stephanianum Willd.* and safflower 15 grams each; *Resina Draconis* 9 grams; spirits 2, 500 grams; sugar 1, 000 grams.

Pharmaceutical Process:

Make medicated spirit from them.

Actions:

Dispels wind and dampness and dredges the channels and collaterals to promote the flow of blood and *qi*.

Indications:

Arthralgia due to wind, cold and dampness, hemiparalysis, malignant sore, scabies and pellagra.

Administration and Dosage:

Oral administration, 15ml. for adults 2 — 3 time per day. Children can take smaller doses according to their conditions.

Caution:

Pregnant women must not take it.

Source:

Pharmacopoeia of Preparations of Chinese Medicine

86. *Baxian* Spirit

Ingredients:

Sichuan aconite root, wild aconite root, peppermint, baked ginger, Chinese angelica root, bamboo leaves, dried orange peel and licorice root 30 grams each; spirits and vinegar 500 grams each; brown sugar 1, 000 grams.

Pharmaceutical Process:

Make medicated spirit of them.

Actions:

Dispels wind and cold, relaxes the muscles and tendons and promotes blood circulation.

Indications:

Arthralgia due to wind, cold and dampness, hemiparalysis (with symptoms of numbness of the limbs, stiffness and spasm of the joints, difficulty in stretching the limbs, pains in the limbs, hemiparalysis, distortion of the eyes and mouth and dysphasis).

Administration and Dosage:

Oral administration, 10—20ml doses, twice per day before meals.

Cautions:

Do not take medicine containing rhinoceros horn, fritillary bulb, fruit-rind of Chinese trichosanthes, tuber of pinellia, bletilla tuber and ampelopsis root while taking the spirit; pregnant women must not take it.

Source:

Practical Preparations in *Pharmacopoeia of Preparations of Chinese Medicine*, 1991, p. 223.

87. Rheumatism Spirit

Ingredients:

Spirits 8, 000 grams, sugar 800 grams, rice fermented with red yeast 32 grams; Chinese angelica root, fruit of Chinese flowering quince, rhizome of cyathula, bark of eucommia (parched with salt), large-leaved gentian, teasel root, leafy stem of Chinese starjasmine, *Morinda officinalis* (prepared), rhizome of *Homalomena occulata*, *Schizophragma intergrifolium Oliv. Phryma leptostachya var. asiatica*, ephedra twig, cinnamom twig, Sichuan aconite root (prepared), wild aconite root (prepared), common St. Paulswort 18 grams each; rhizome of Ligusticum Chuanxiong, dried orange peel, sandalwood, fingered citron fruit 12 grams each; licorice root and rhizome of birthwood 9 grams each.

Pharmaceutical Process:

Make medicated spirit of them.

Actions:

Dispels wind and cold and dredges the channels and collaterals to promote blood circulafion.

Indications:

Arthralgia due to wind, cold and dampness (with symptoms of numbness of the limbs, pains in the waist and legs and difficulty in walking).

Administration and Dosage:

30—50ml doses, 3 times per day.

Cautions:

Do not take medicine containing rhinoceros horn, fritillary bulb, fruit-rind of Chinese trichosanthes, tuber of pinellia, bletilla tuber and ampelopsis root while taking the spirit; pregnant women must not take it.

Source:

Proved Recipes in *Practical Preparations of Chinese Medicine*, 1991, p. 223.

Section Eleven   Traumatic Injury

Traumatic injury is common and its clinical symptoms are local blood stasis, swelling and pains or restriction of motion.

1. Spirit for Traumatic Injury and Rheumatism

Ingredients:

Root of ledang 45 grams, rose root 45 grams, rhizome of *Lindera glauca Bl*. 24 grams.

Pharmaceutical Process:

Soak the herbs in 50 grams of 50% proof spirit for half a month.

Actions:

Dispels wind and dampness and promotes blood circulation to relieve pain.

Indications:

Sudden sprain and contusion, rheumatic arthritis and lumbar muscle strain.

Administration and Dosage:

Oral administration for sudden sprain and contusion twice per day, 100ml dose the first time and 50ml each time later. Also apply topically. For lumbar muscle strain and rheumatic arthritis, 50ml doses, twice per day. 20 days constitute a course of treatment. The patient with serious inflammation of injury should have 2 courses of treatment. If he has a dry and hot throat during the treatment, he can discontinue taking the spirit and resume the therapy a few days later.

Source:

Medical, Scientific and Technical Materials, Issue 2, 1972,

p. 17.

2. Spirit for Sprain

Ingredients:

Cassia bark 2. 4 grams, Sichuan aconite root 36 grams, safflower 2. 4 grams, wild aconite root 36 grams, perilla stem 60 grams, ledebouriella root 36 grams, ephedra twig 60 grams, rhizome of birthwood 36 grams, giant typhonium tuber 60 grams, frankincense 36 grams, *Lycopodium clavatum L.* 60 grams, myrrh 36 grams, *Lycopodium casuarinoides Spring* 60 grams, Tiantai aconite root 36 grams, futokadsura stem 60 grams, *Caulis Clematidis Amandii* 36 grams, root of Chinese climatis 60 grams, Chinese angelica root 48 grams, *Vitex trifolia* 60 grams, root of slender acanthopanax 96 grams, *Schizonepeta tenuifolia* 36 grams, spirits 7,000 grams, achyranthes root 60 grams, root of Ligusticum Chuanxiong 48 grams.

Pharmaceutical Process:

Mix the herbs well and infuse them twice in the spirit by submerging them in part of the spirit and letting them infuse for 7 days, stirring them periodically. Filtrate them, add the remaining spirit to the dregs, let them infuse for over 3 days, stirring them periodically. Then filtrate them and mix the two filtrates.

Actions:

Dissipates blood stasis and promotes blood circulation and activates the flow of *qi* to relieve pain.

Indications:

Traumatic injury.

Administration and Dosage:

Apply topically to the affected part.

Caution:

Do not take it orally.

Source:

Common Methods of Making up Prescriptions of Chinese and Western Medicine, ed. The No. 1 People's Pharmaceutical Factory of Chengdu, 1973.

3. Spirit of Safflower

Ingredients:

Safflower 100 grams.

Pharmaceutical Process:

Let the safflower infuse in 1,000ml of spirits for 7 days, then filtrate it. Keep the filtrate static at room temperature for 48 hours, filtrate it again and pack the filtrate separately in 100—200ml bottles.

Actions:

Promotes blood circulation to relieve pain.

Indications:

Traumatic injury and rheumatic arthritis.

Administration and Dosage:

Oral administration, 10ml doses, twice per day.

Source:

Beihe Production Brigade of Daqinggua Commune of Tieling County, *Liaonining Medicine*, Supplementary Issue 2, 1975, p. 28.

4. Spirit of Japanese Yam

Ingredient:

Japanese yam 600 grams.

Pharmaceutical Process:

Cut the yam into slices and let them infuse in 1, 000ml of 50% proof spirits for 15 days. Filtrate the infusion, keep the filtrate static at room temperature for 48 hours, then filtrate it and pack the filtrate separately in 100—200ml bottles.

Actions:

Relaxes the muscles and tendons and promotes blood circulation to relieve pain.

Indications:

Traumatic injury, waist sprain and rheumatism, etc.

Administration and Dosage:

Oral administration, 10ml doses, twice per day.

Source:

Liaoning Medicine, Supplementary Issue 2, 1975

5. Spirit for Traumatic Injury

Ingredients:

Bupleurum root 12 grams, teasel root 6 grams, Chinese angelica root 12 grams, nux-vomica seed (without villus) 6 grams, rhizome of Ligusticum Chuanxiong 12 grams, drynaria rhizome (without villus) 6 grams, scutellaria root 6 grams, safflower 4 grams, peach kernels 6 grams, buried tuber 4 grams, trogopterus dung 6 grams, frankincense (prepared with vinegar) 3 grams, red peony root 6 grams, spirit of 60% alcohol cortent 1, 000 ml., sappan wood 6 grams.

Pharmaceutical Process:

Grind the herbs into small pieces, mix them well, put them into a bag and tie up the mouth. Let the herbs infuse airtight in the spirit for about 30 days, then press them, filtrate them, keep the filtrate static to settle the dregs and pack the clear liquid in bottles.

Actions:

Relaxes the muscles and tendons, promotes blood circulation and subdues swelling to relieve pain.

Indications:

Traumatic injury, blood stasis, lingering swelling and stiffness of the muscles and tendons and obstruction in the channels and collaterals.

Administration and Dosage:

Oral administration 30—60ml doses, twice per day. Or apply topically.

Remarks:

The prescription of the spirit for traumatic injury in *Pharmacy* of the Pharmaceutical department of Jiangxi Medicinal College is similar to the prescription mentioned above in ingredients, but different from it in preparation method. The process of the former is to grind the herbs together, mix them well and wet the mixture with 56% proof spirits. First, let it infuse in this kind of spirits for 72 hours according to the method of percolation, then percolate the infusion at a speed of 1-3ml per minute. Add the simple syrup made of 120 grams of brown sugar to the percolate, mix them well and keep the mixture static for some time. Finally, filtrate it and pack it.

Source:

Pharmacy and Annotations to Preparations, Fascicle 3, Vol. 2, ed. Department of Pharmacy of Beijing Medical College, 1976.

6. Spirit for Traumatic Injury

Ingredients:

Chinese angelica root, rhizome of slender acanthopanax and rhizome of rehmannia 30 grams each; psoralea fruit, drynaria rhzome, leaf of *Mahonia bealei*, seed of Job's tears and root bark of *Cercis chinensis Bge*, 15 grams each; rhizome of birthwood, noterpterygium root, rhizome of zedoary and peach kernels 9 grams each; rhizome of Ligusticum Chuanxiong and eucommia bark 24 grams; tiger bone (crisp fried in a liquid) 36 grams, spirits 10,000 grams.

Pharmaceutical Process:

Put the ingredients into a jar, seal it up, put it into a larger container with water and decoct the ingredients for the time it takes to burn 3 joss sticks. Drink it 7 days later.

Indication:

Traumatic injury.

Administration and Dosage:

Twice per day, in the morning and the evening.

Source:

Encyclopaedia of Surgeons, *Vol.* 36

7. Spirit of *Claoxylon Polot Merr*.

Ingredients:

Bark of *Claoxylon polot Merr*. 2 portions, *Centipeda minima* 2 portions, shandayang 1 portion, magufeng 1 portion, *Piper boehmeriaefolium Wall. var. Tonkinense C. DC.* 1 portion, kuanjinteng 1 portion, *Penthorum chinense Pursh* 1 portion, *Viscum articulatum Brrm. f.* 1 portion, coriander 1 portion, *Uncaria rhynchophylla* 1 portion, resticulate 1 portion, short-petalled China pink 1 portion, *Ranunculus japonicus Thunb*. 1 portion.

Pharmaceutical Process:

Submerge the herbs in millet wine of 50—60% alcohol content, and let them infuse for over 7 days, or for 2 days in hot millet wine.

Actions:

Relaxes the muscles and tendons, promotes blood circulation and dispels wind to relieve pain.

Indications:

Traumatic injury, bone fracture, sprain, joint stiffness, acute and chronic rheumatic arthritis, rheumatic heart disease, sciatica, rheumatoid arthritis, muscular rheumatism, bone tuberculosis, hyperosteogeny, arthroncus of the knee, pains in the waist and legs, child paralysis, etc.

Administration and Dosage:

Topical application or oral administration, 15-30ml doses or 50ml doses if the disease is serious, 2-3 times per day.

Caution:

Pregnant women must not take it because *Claoxylon polot Merr and Penthorum chinense Pursh* and reticulate are abortifacients.

Source:

News of Hygiene in Brief, Issue 5-6, ed. Bureau of Public Health of Baizou Prefecture, Guangxi, 1977, p. 74.

8. Spirit of Safflower

Ingredients:

Liaoning safflower and garden balsam 50 grams each; alum q. s.

Pharmaceutical Process:

Let the ingredients infuse in 1,000 grams of spirits of 60% alcohol cortent for 24 hours and filtrate the infusion.

Actions:

Subdues swelling to relieve pain.

Indication:

Traumatic injury.

Administration and Dosage:

Let a piece of gauze infuse in the filtrate for 20 minutes and apply it to the affected part, keeping it wet. Once per day or every other day.

Source:

Chinese Medicine of Liaoning, Trial Issue, 1977.

9. Spirit of Drynaria

Ingredients:

Drynaria rhizome 60 grams, spirits 500 grams.

Pharmaceutical Process:

Let the herb infuse in the spirit for 7 days.

Indications:

Traumatic injury, bone fracture.

Administration and Dosage:

Oral administration, 10ml doses, twice per day or topical application (for alopecia areata).

Source:

Chinese Medicated Dietetics, 1985, p. 228.

10. Spirit of *Ophisaurus Harti Boulenger*

Ingredients:

Ophisaurus harti Boulenger, spirits 500 grams.

Pharmaceutical Process:

Let the snake infuse in the spirit for 7 days.

Actions:

Dissipates blood stasis, dispels wind, subdues swelling and relieves intoxication.

Indications:

Arthralgia due to wind and cold, traumatic injury and bone fracture.

Administration and Dosage:

10ml, doses, twice per day

Source:

Chinese Medicated Dietetics, 1985, p. 257.

11. Spirit of Pseudo-Ginseng

Ingredients:

Pseudo-ginseng 10-30 grams, spirits 500 grams.

Pharmaceutical Process:

Let the herb infuse in the spirit for 7 days.

Actions:

Promotes blood circulation, stops bleeding and subdues swelling to relieve pain.

Indications:

Traumatic injury and pain due to blood stasis.

Administration and Dosage:

5-10ml doses, 2-3 times per day.

Source:

Chinese Medicated Dietetics, 1985, p. 258.

12. Spirit of Chinese Flowering Quince

Ingredients:

Fruit of Chinese flowering quince 15 grams; rhizome of slender acanthopanax, sargentgloryvine, rhizome of Chinese climatis, 12 grams each.

Pharmaceutical Process:

Grind the herbs and take the powder with hot millet wine.

Indications:

Traumatic injury, lumbago and foot pain.

Adminstration and Dosage:

6 gram doses, twice per day.

Source:

A Handbook of Family Dietetic Therapy, 1982, p. 173.

13. Spirit of Chinese Flowering Quince

Ingredients:

Fruit of Chinese flowering quince, yellow millet wine *q. s.*

Pharmaceutical Process:

Decoct the fruit in the wine.

Indications:

Spasm of the calf muscle.

Administration and Dosage:

10ml before sleep till recovery.

Source:

A Handbook of Family Dietetic Therapy, 1982, p. 174.

14. Spirit of Sheep Tibia

Ingredients:

Sheep tibia, spirits *q. s.*

Pharmaceutical Process:

Break up the tibia and let the pieces infuse in the spirit for 7 days.

Indication:

Spasm and pain of the muscles, tendons and bones.

Administration and Dosage:

Twice per day and 10ml. each time.

Source:

A Handbook of Family Dietetic Therapy, 1982, p. 195.

15. Spirit of Drynaria

Ingredients:

Drynaria rhizome 720 grams, yellow millet wine 500 grams.

Pharmaceutical Process:

Let the herb infuse in the wine for 7 days.

Indications:

Traumatic injury and bone fracture.

Administration and Dosage:

30ml doses, twice per day. The dregs can be ground into small pieces, dried and applied topically to heal a fracture.

Source:

Compendium Medica of Guangzhou

16. Wine of Crabs

Ingredients:

A male and female live freshwater crab, mellow millet wine 1,000 grams.

Pharmaceutical Process:

Decoct the crabs in the wine for half an hour and use the wine for treatment.

Indication:

Pain due to traumatic injury.

Administration and Dosage:

Divide the wine into 3 doses and sleep soundly for 2 hours

after taking each dose.

Source:

Journal of Chinese Medicine of Jiangsu

17. Wine of Fingered Citron

Ingredients:

Fruit of fingered citron prepared with vinegar 15 grams, millet wine 30 grams, water *q. s.*

Pharmaceutical Process:

Decoct the fruit in the wine.

Indications:

Pain due to traumatic injury.

Administration and Dosage:

Take it while it is hot.

Source:

Medicinal Fruits

18. Spirit of Spatholobus

Ingredients:

Spatholobus stem and rock candy 60 grams each; spirits 500 grams.

Pharmaceutical Process:

Let the herb and candy infuse in the spirit for 7 days.

Indication:

Traumatic injury.

Administration and Dosage:

15-20ml doses, twice per day.

Source:

1,100 *Folk Prescriptions of Dietetic Therapy*, 1992, p. 193.

19. Dali Spirit

Ingredients:

Rhizome of *Salvia miltiorrhiza Bge.* , Chinese angelica root, safflower, root of Dahurian angelica, Sichuan aconite root, frankincense, myrrh, rhizome of rhubarb, root of herbaceous peony, drynaria rhizome, *Ophisaurus harti Boulenger*, green tangerine peel, teasel root, burreed tuber, *curcuma zedoaria*, rhizome of rehmannia, pseudo-ginseng, rhizome of slender acanthopanax, achyranthes root, native copper, ground beetle, madder root, spirit.

Pharmaceutical Process:

Let the snake, herbs, beetle and copper infuse in the spirit.

Actions:

Relaxes the muscles and tendons, dispels wind and dampness and promotes blood circulation to relieve pain.

Indications:

Traumatic injury and arthralgia due to wind, cold and dampness.

Administration and Dosage:

5-10ml doses for slight and new injury and 10-20ml for serious and old injury 3 times per day.

Cautions:

Pregnant women must not take it and debilitated patients should be cautious in taking it.

Storage:

Keep it airtight in a dark and cool place.

Source:

A Practical Handbook of Prepared Chinese Medicine, 1985, p. 110.

Section Twelve   Protrusion of Intervertebral Disc

Protrusion intervertebral disc is a common disease. Because of its own decay or extrinsic pressure, the intervertebral disc protrudes backward and presses the nerve roots, thus causing radiation pain in the nerves and their dysfunction.

1. Spirit of Rhododendron Molle

Ingredients:

Rhizome of Rhododendron molle and rhizome of rehmannia 500 grams each; spatholobus stem 250 grams, cinnamom twig 200 grams, spirits 5,000 grams.

Pharmaceutical Process:

Sprinkle the herbs with cold boiled water and let them infuse in the spirits for 7 days.

Indication:

Protrusion of intervertebral disc.

Administration and Dosage:

Oral administration. At first, 10ml doses, 3 times per day; later, increase the dosage gradually till slight numbness is felt in the limbs, Keep to this dosage for a week and reduce it gradually.

Remarks:

Take atropine should side effects of nausea, vomiting and a reduction in heart rate occur. Mainly use the rhizome of the herb to treat rheumatic arthralgia and myalgia, for it is not so poisonous as the flowers, which are highly toxic and can be lethal if used improperly.

Section Thirteen   Lumbago Due to Renal Deficiency

Lumbago refers to the pain in one side or both sides of the lower part of the back. Lumbago has much to do with the kidneys, whose deficiency is its major cause.

1. Spirit of Deer Bone

Ingredients:

Deer bone 100 grams, eucommia bark and Sichuan teasel root 9 grams each, spirits 1,000 grams.

Pharmaceutical Process:

Let the bone and herbs infuse in the spirit for 10 days.

Indications:

Soreness and weakness of the waist and knees induced by the deficiency of the kidneys and injury of the muscles, tendons and bones.

Administration and Dosage:

10ml doses, twice per day.

Source:

Chinese Medicated Dietetics, 1985, p. 302.

2. Spirit of Pig Kidney

Ingredients:

One pig kidney, two cups of the urine of a boy under 12, one wine glass of spirits.

Pharmaceutical Process:

Put the ingredients into an earthenware bottle, seal it up with mud and begin decocting the ingredients in the evening. Open the bottle before dawn and take them.

Indication:

Lumbago due to renal deficiency.

Administration and Dosage:

Eat the kidney and drink the spirit.

Source:

Fei Boxiong (in the Qing Dynasty), *Materia Medica.*

3. Spirit of *Epimedium Brevicornum and Spatholobus*

Ingredients:

Epimedium brevicornum E. koreanum, morinda root, spatholobus stem 30 grams each; spirits 1,000 grams, rock candy 60 grams.

Pharmaceutical Process:

Let the herbs infuse in the spirit for 7 days.

Indications:

Rheumatic pains in the waist and legs and lumbago caused by renal deficiency.

Administration and Dosage:

Oral administration.

Source:

Chinese Medicated Dietetics, 1985, p, 222.

4. Spirit of Dogwood

Ingredients:

Dogwood fruit 30-50 grams, spirit 500 grams.

Pharmaceutical Process:

Let the fruit infuse in the spirit for 7 days.

Indications:

Lumbago due to renal deficiency, spermatorrhea, general weakness and hyperhidrosis.

Administration and Dosage:

10-20ml doses, once or twice per day.

Source:

Chinese Medicated Dietetics, 1985, p, 220.

5. Spirit of Jujube Fruit

Ingredients:

Walnut kernels, jujube fruit and honey 60 grams each; almonds and butter 30 grams, spirits 750 grams.

Pharmaceutical Process:

melt the honey and butter and mix them with the spirit. Grind the other three ingredients, add them to the spirits, put them into a bottle and keep the bottle airtight for 21 days.

Indications:

Lumbago due to renal deficiency.

Source:

Nourishment Therapy

Section Fourteen   Lumber Sprain

Lumbar sprain often takes place in the loin and can affect the muscles, ligaments, fasciae, small intervertebral joints, lumbosacral joints or sacro-iliac articulations. The sprained part is painful and tender.

1. Spirit of *Shenqu*

Ingredient:

shenqu (fermented mix of flour, bran, almonds, wormwood) 1 piece as big as a fist.

Pharmaceutical Process:

Heat *shenqu* till it turns red, then put it into 2 big cups of spirit and drink it immediately.

Indication:

Lumbar sprain.

Administration and Dosage:

Drink up the spirit and lie on back for a short while.

Source:

Effective Prescriptions, *Vol.* 3

2. Spirit of Antler

Ingredient:

Antler newly-cut, 2—3 *cun* long and heated red hot.

Pharmaceutical Process:

Let it infuse in spirit for 2 days.

Indication:

Lumbago and difficluty in turning around or turning over.

Administration and Dosage:

Oral administration before meals.

Source:

Essentials of Diet, Vol. 2, *Dietectic Therapy*.

3. Wine of Chinese Chives

Ingredients:

Chinese chives or their roots 30 grams, yellow millet wine 100 grams.

Pharmaceutical Process:

Cut the chives into thin strips and heat them with the wine.

Administration and Dosage:

Oral administration once or twice per day.

Source:

Chinese Dietetic Therapy, p. 304.

Section Fifteen   Cervical Disease

Cervical disease refers to cervical retrograde degeneration, the major symptom of which is cervical and shoulder pains which can radiate to the forearms and hands when the cervical nerve roots are pressed. If the disease is serious, it can result in the decline of the dermal sensation and the muscualr atrophia of the affected part.

1. Spirit of Egg Plant Peel and Antler

Ingredients:

Egg plant peel 120 grams, pilose antler 60 grams, spirits 500 ml.

Pharmaceutical Process:

Let the peel and antler infuse in the spirit for 7 days, remove the dregs, filtrate the infusion and add some brown sugar.

Indication:

Cervical disease.

Administration and Dosage:

Oral administration, 2-3 times per day.

Source:

Chinese Dietetic Therapy, p. 303.

Section Sixteen   Obstruction of Qi in the Chest

The major symptoms of obstruction of *qi* in the chest are chest pain, which sometimes even radiates to the whole back, short breath and asthma, which makes even reclining impossible. It is similar to coronary heart disease in modern medicine.

1. Spirit of Snakegourd and Macrostem Onion

Ingredients:

Snakegourd fruit 12 grams, macrostem onion 9 grams, spirits *q. s.*

Pharmaceutical Process:

Decoct the ingredients together or with water.

Actions:

Activates *yang*, removes obstruction, promotes the flow of *qi* and removes the phlegm.

Indications:

Obstruction of *qi* in the chest (with symptoms of vague chest pain, bad chest pain radiating to the whole back, asthma, cough, white and moist fur on the tongue and deep pulse).

Administration and Dosage:

Oral administration, once or twice daily.

Source:

Synopsis of Prescriptions of the Golden Chamber

2. Wine of Sheep Blood

Ingredients:

Half a bowl of fresh sheep blood, one bowl of millet wine.

Pharmaceutical Process:

Heat the wine till it boils, add the blood and mix them well.

Indication:

Acute cardialgia.

Administration and Dosage:

Take it at a draught or at two draughts.

Source:

A Handbook of Family Dietetic Therapy, 1982, p. 191.

3. Spirit of Red Sage

Ingredients:

Red sage root 30 grams, spirits 500 grams.

Pharmaceutical Process:

Let the root infuse in the spirit for 7 days.

Indication:

Pain due to blood stasis and obstruction in the channels and collaterals.

Administration and Dosage:

20-30ml doses, 2-3 times per day.

Source:

Chinese Medicated Dietetics, 1985, p. 263.

4. Spirit of Glossy Ganoderma and Red Sage

Ingredients:

Glossy ganoderma 30 grams, red sage root 50 grams, pseudo-ginseng 15 grams, spirits 500 grams.

Pharmaceutical Process:

Let glossy ganoderma, red sage root and pseudo-ginseng infuse in spirits for 7 days.

Indication:

Coronary heart disease.

Administration and Dosage:

20-30ml doses, twice per day.

Source:

1,100 *Folk Prescriptions of Dietetic Therapy*, 1992, p. 57.

Section Seventeen   Headache

Headache is a common and conscious symptom that may occur alone and in various kinds of acute and chronic diseases.

1. Wine of Fermented Soybeans

Ingredients:

Fermented soybeans 15 grams, scallion root 30 grams, yellow millet wine 50 ml.

Pharmaceutical Process:

Decoct the soybeans in water for 10 minutes, add the scallion root, decoct them for 50 minutes and add the wine.

Indication:

Headache.

Administration and Dosage:

Take it at a draught while it is still hot.

Source:

Chinese Dietetic Therapy, p. 377.

2. Wine of Chrysanthemum

Ingredients:

Chrysanthemum flowers 100 grams, Chinese wolfberry fruit 100 grams, Shaoxing wine *q. s.*

Pharmaceutical Process:

Let the flowers and fruit infuse in the wine for 10-20 days, remove the dregs, filtrate the infusion and add some honey.

Indications:

Lingering wind syndrome of the head, headache and dizziness.

Administration and Dosage:

10ml in the morning and evening.

Source:

Food, Chinese Medicine and Folk Prescriptions.

3. Spirit of Ox Brains

Ingredients:

Ox brains, slices of root of Dahurian angelica and ground root of Ligusticum Chuanxiong 9 grams each.

Pharmaceutical Process:

Put the ingredients into a magnetic container and decoct them with spirit.

Indications:

Wind syndrome of the head.

Administration and Dosage:

Take it while it is hot and go to sleep after that.

Source:

A Handbook of Family Dietetic Therapy, 1982, p. 509.

4. Spirit of *Ligusticum Chuanxiong*

Ingredients:

Root of Ligusticum Chuanxiong 30 grams, spirits 500 grams.

Pharmaceutical Process:

Let the root infuse in the spirits for 7 days.

Indication:

Pain due to traumatic injury and wind syndrome of the head.

Administration and Dosage:

10—20ml doses, 2—3 times per day.

Source:

Chinese Medicated Dietetics, 1985, p. 264.

Section Eighteen   Vertigo

Vertigo or dizziness may stop when the patient closes his

142

eyes if it is slight. If it is serious, the patient will feel as if he were riding a train or a boat, everything is spinning round, unable to stand, and will have nausea and vomiting at the same time.

1. Spirit of Eucommia

Ingredients:

Eucommia bark 30 grams, spirits 500 grams.

Pharmaceutical Process:

Let the bark infuse in the spirit for 7 days.

Indications:

Hypertension and lumbago caused by strain.

Administration and Dosage:

10—20ml doses, 2—3 times per day.

Source:

Chinese Medicated Dietetics, 1985, p. 223.

2. Wine of Chinese Yam

Ingredients:

Chinese yam, dogwood fruit, fruit of Chinese magnoliavine, ginseng.

Pharmaceutical Process:

Decoct the ingredients in millet wine or spirit.

Indications:

Dizziness due to the wind syndrome of the head.

Administration and Dosage:

Oral administration.

Source:

A Handbook of Family Dietetic Therapy, 1982, p. 513.

3. Wine of Chrysanthemum

Ingredient:

White chrysanthemum flowers 60 grams.

Pharmaceutical Process:

Mince the flowers and let them infuse in wine for 7 days.

Administration and Dosage:

Dizziness, headache and conjunctival congestion.

Administration and Dosage:

30ml doses, twice per day.

Source:

A Dictionary of Chinese Medicine

Section Nineteen   Apoplexy

The major symptoms of apoplexy are distortion of the eyes and mouth, hemiparalysis and slurred speech, concomitant with or without sudden syncope and loss of consciousness.

1. *Shiguogong* Spirit

Ingredients:

Chinese angelica root, tiger tibia (infused for a day, baked and stir-fried in a liquid to make it crisp), noterpterygium root, freshwater turtle shell (stir-fried in a liquid), *Dioscorea hypoglauce*, ledebouriella root, large-leaved gentian, rhizome of cyathula, nodular branch of pine and silkworm excrement 60 grams each; Chinese wolfberry fruit 150 grams, dried eggplant root (steamed) 240 grams.

Pharmaceutical Process:

Put the ingredients into a silk bag and let them infuse airtight in one decalitre of limeless wine for 10 days.

Indications:

Hemiparalysis, lingering numbness of the limbs, arthralgia

144

due to wind, cold and dampness.

Administration and Dosage:

Oral administration, twice per day in the morning and evening.

Source:

Standards of Diagnosis and Treatment, Vol. 1.

2. Spirit of Black-Bone Hen

Ingredients:

Black-bone hen (cleaned).

Pharmaceutical Process:

Boil the hen with 2,500ml of spirits down to 1,000ml. Remove the dregs, divide the remaining spirits into 3 doses and take them one after another.

Indications:

Apoplexy, stiffness of the back, aphasia caused by the rigidity of the tongue, failure in rolling the eyes and dysphoria with a suffocated feeling.

Source:

Essentials of Diet, Vol. 2, *Dietetic Therapy* (written in the Yuan Dynasty).

3. *Linru* Spirit

Ingredients:

Wild aconite root 750 grams; Chinese angelica root, galangal rhizome and cloves 250 grams each.

Pharmaceutical Process:

Grind the cloves into small pieces, cut the remainig herbs into slices, mix them, put them into a bag, add 6,000ml of spirits of 60% alcohol content and tie the mouth. Steam the ingredients to make the internal temperature of the bag reach 65-70℃ and maintain the temperature for 24 hours. Then reduce the heat to room temperature, filtrate the ingredients, press the dregs and mix the extract with the filtrate. Stir-fry 1,000 grams of brown sugar till the sugar turns dark brown and tastes bitter, then mix it with the medicated spirits. Keep the mixture static for 5-7 days, filtrate it with gauze to obtain clear extract and pack it.

Actions:

Warms the middle-*jiao*, promotes blood circulation and dispels wind and cold.

Indications:

Rheumatic numbness, cold and pain in the back, hemiparalysis, distortion of the eyes and mouth and puerperal apoplexy.

Administration and Dosage:

Oral administration, 1ml doses before breakfast and supper.

Cautions:

Do not eat very hot food within 2 hours after taking it; pregnant women and hypertension and heart patients must not take it. Drink half a bowl of cold boiled water with 1 *liang* of brown sugar should side effects of dizziness, nausea and general numbness and weakness occur.

Source:

Medicinal Criteria of Henan Province, 1977.

4. Ginger Spirit

Ingredient:

Ginger.

Pharmaceutical Process:

Let the ginger infuse in spirits.

Indications:

Migraine due to wind, nausea, chronic infectious disease and cold and pain in the abdomen and scrobiculus cordis.

Administration and Dosage:

Oral administration, 300ml while it is warm.

Source:

A Handbook of Family Dietetic Therapy, 1982, p. 514.

5. Spirit of Black-Tail Snake

Ingredients:

Zaocys dhumnades, spirits 500 grams.

Pharmaceutical Process:

Let the snake infuse in the spirit for 7 days.

Indications:

Arthralgia due to wind and dampness, difficulty in stretching the limbs and hemiparalysis.

Administration and Dosage:

10ml. doses, twice per day.

Source:

Chinese Medicated Dietetics, 1985, p. 256.

6. Spirit of *Agkistrodon Acutus*

Ingredients:

Agkistrodon acutus, spirits 500 grams.

Pharmaceutical Process:

Let the snake infuse in the spirit for 7 days.

Indications:

Arthralgia due to wind and dampness, difficulty in stretching the limbs and hemiparalysis.

7. Spirit of *Poncirus Trifolia*

Ingredient:

Fruit of *Poncirus trifolia*.

Pharmaceutical Process:

Let the fruit infuse in the spirit.

Indications:

General rigidity caused by apoplexy and distortion of the eyes and mouth.

Administration and Dosage:

Oral administration.

Source:

A Handbook of Family Dietetic Therapy, 1982, p. 515.

8. Black Soybeans Sprinkled with Spirit

Ingredient:

Black soybeans.

Pharmaceutical Process:

Parch the beans till they get crisp and sprinkle them with spirit.

Benefits:

Dissipates blood stasis and dispels wind.

Indications:

Men's apoplexy, distortion of the eyes and mouth, abdominal pain and hematuria, women's diseases induced by puerperal apoplexy.

Administration and Dosage:

Drink it while it is warm.

Source:

A Handbook of Family Dietetic Therapy, 1982, p. 516.

9. Wine of Black Soybeans

148

Ingredients:

Black soybeans 500 grams, millet wine 3,000 grams.

Pharmaceutical Process:

Put the beans and spirits into a jar, seal it up and put it over a slow charcoal fire. Remove the beans when half of the spirit is left.

Indication:

Sequelae of apoplexy.

Administration and Dosage:

20ml. each time.

Source:

General Collection of Prescriptions for Holy Relief

10. Wine of Gastrodia

Ingredients:

Gastrodia tuber, achyranthes root and parched eucommia bark 24 grams, yellow millet wine 1,000 grams.

Pharmaceutical Process:

Cut the herbs into small pieces, put them into a bag and let them infuse in the wine for 7 days.

Actions:

Calms the endopathic wind and relieves spasms.

Indications:

Numbness of the limbs and difficulty in stretching the hands and feet.

Administration and Dosage:

10ml. doses, twice per day.

Source:

Effective Prescriptions.

Section Twenty   Flaccidity Syndrome

Flaccidity syndrome refers to the muscular atrophia of the limbs, which eventually induces their debilitation and disablement. At the onset of the disease, the patient feels weakness in his lower limbs and then in his hands and feet. At last, his muscles become numb and his skin loses lustre and dries up.

1. Pills of Spirit and Achyranthes

Ingredients:

Achyranthes root (stir-fried in a liquid till it turns yellow) 90 grams; Sichuan pepper and tiger bone (stir-fried in vinegar till it turns yellow) 15 grams each; stir-baked aconite root.

Pharmaceutical Process:

Grind them all into small pieces, put them into a silk bag and let them infuse in one decalitre of decocted spirits (for 10 days in spring and autumn, for 7 days in summer and for 14 days in winter). Mix the dregs with vinegar and make the mixture into pills.

Indications:

Soreness and weakness of the muscles, tendons and bones of the waist and feet.

Administration and Dosage:

Oral administration, 20ml. of the spirits before meals every day and 20-30 pills with warm spirits or salt water before meals every day.

Source:

A Dictionary of Chinese Medicine

2. Spirit of Tiger Bone

Ingredients:

Tiger bone (stir-fried in a liquid) 150 grams, red sage root 60 grams, root of Chinese wolfberry; dried ginger and rhizome of Ligusticum Chuanxiong 30 grams each; prepared rhizome of rehmannia 30. 9 grams; rhizome of slender acanthopanax, fruit of *Poncirus trifoliata* (parched with bran) and rhizome of large-headed atractylodes 30. 3 grams each.

Pharmaceutical Process:

Grind the ingredients into small pieces, put them into a silk bag and let them infuse in 4 decalitres of mellow spirit for 4 days.

Indications:

Arthralgia, spasm and contracture of the tendons, overstrain, deficiency of and cold in the liver and bitter taste and dysphoria.

Administration and Dosage:

Oral administration, twice per day; 2-3 decalitres the first time and 1 small cup before meals later.

Source:

Prescriptions Assigned to the Three Categories of Pathogenic Factors of Disease. Vol. 8

3. Spirit of *Sesamum Indicum DC*.

Ingredients:

Seed of *Sesamum indicum DC*. 100 grams, seed of Job's tears 30 grams, dired root of rehmannia 250 grams, spirits 1,000 grams.

Pharmaceutical Process:

Put the seed and root into a silk bag and let them infuse in the spirit for 3-5 days, shaking them frequently.

Actions:

Strengthens the muscles, tendons and bones and dispels wind and dampness.

Indications:

Deficiency of the liver and the kidneys, malnutrition of the muscles, tendons and bones; weakness of the waist and knees due to rheumatic arthralgia; and muscle and tendon spasms that induce sharp pain.

Storage:

Keep it airtight in a dark and cool place.

Source:

A Handbook of Dietetic Physicians

4. Spirit of Finest Cream

Ingredients:

100ml of finest cream.

Pharmaceutical Process:

Mix the cream with spirit.

Actions:

Dispels wind and dampness.

Indications:

Weakness and deficiency.

Administration and Dosage:

Drink it while it is warm.

Source:

Essentials of Diet, Dietectic Therapy.

5. Spirit of Nodular Branch of Pine

Ingredient:

Nodular branch of pine (gathered on May 5).

Pharmaceutical Process:

Break it up and make medicated spirit with it.

Indications:

Deficiency of the bones and weakness of the feet.

Source:

Essentials of Diet, Vol. 3, *Spirit*.

6. Spirit of Slender Acanthopanax

Ingredient:

Rhizome of slender acanthopanax.

Pharmaceutical Process:

Let the rhizome infuse in spirits.

Indication:

Debilitation of the bones.

Source:

Essentials of Diet, Vol. 3, Spirit.

7. Spirit of Ginseng and Antler

Ingredients:

Pilose antler, ginseng, achyranthes root, prepared rhizome of rehmannia, desertliving cistanche stem, dodder seed, prepared aconite root, astragalus root, fruit of chinese magnoliavine, *Poria cocos*, Chinese yam, Chinese angelica root, fossil fragments, root of narrow-leaved polygala, rice fermented with red yeast.

Actions:

Nourishes the kindneys, strengthens *yang* and controls nocturnal emission.

Indications:

Flaccidity syndrome including soreness and weakness of the waist and knees, difficulty in walking, cold hands and feet, muscular atrophia and disablement of the limbs, spermatorrhea which induces lumbago, impotence, premature ejeculation, pale face, weakness of the limbs, lassitude, sterility; deep, thready and weak pulse and pale tongue with white fur; leukorrhagia with white thin, profuse leukorrhea without stink; vague pain in the lower part of the abdomen, lumbago and weak and cold limbs.

Administration and Dosage:

Oral administration, 6—9ml doses, twice per day.

Caution:

Those who have a fever must not take it.

Source:

Medicinal Standards of Heilongjiang Province (1980) in *Basic Preparations of Chinese Medicine*, Vol. 1, 1988, p. 236.

8. Spirit of Pine Root Juice

Ingredient:

Pine root juice.

Pharmaceutical Process:

Dig a pit by the roots of a pine tree, gather their juice and make medicated spirit with it.

Indication:

Rheumatism.

Source:

Essentials of Diet, *Spirit*.

9. Gruel of Spirit and Pig Kidneys

Ingredients:

2 pig kidneys, 3 decalitres of glutinous rice, 6 grams of Amomum tsao-ko, 3 grams of dried orange peel.

Pharmaceutical Process:

Remove the fatty membranes of the kidneys, cut them into slices and decoct them with the herbs. Filtrate the thick decoction, remove the dregs, add a little spirits to the filtrate and boil the mixture with the rice.

Indications:

Deficiency and overstrain of the kidneys, weakness of the waist and knees and lumbago.

Administration and Dosage:

Take it before meals.

Source:

Essentials of Diet, Vol. 2, *Dietectic Therapy*.

10. Spirit of Chinese Wolfberry

Ingredient:

Fruit of Ganzhou wolfberry.

Pharmaceutical Process:

Make medicated spirits with it.

Actions:

Restores *qi*, replenishes vital essence, strengthens *yang*, promotes tissue regeneration and dispels cold wind.

Source:

Essentials of Diet, Vol. 3, Spirits.

11. Spirit of Rehmannia

Ingredient:

Rhizome of rehmannia.

Pharmaceutical Process:

Wring juice out of the rhizome and make medicated spirit with it.

Actions:

Restores *qi*, strengthens the muscles, tendons and bones, removes the obstruction in the channels and collaterals and relieves abdominal pain.

Source:

> *Essentials of Diet*, Vol. 3, *Spirit*.

or

Ingredients:

> Dried rhizome of rehmannia 60 grams, spirits 500ml.

Pharmaceutical Process:

> Wash the herb clean, infuse it in the spirits, seal up the bottle, shake it frequently and drink the spirit 7 days later.

Actions:

> Nourishes the blood and promotes blood circulation.

Indications:

> Deficiency of the blood and *yin* and numbness and pains of the limbs induced by malnutrition of the muscles, tendons and channels.

Administration and Dosage:

> Oral administration, 10ml before sleep.

12. Spirit of Achyranthes

Ingredient:

> Achyranthes root.

Pharmaceutical Process:

> Decoct the root and make spirit of its extract and distiller's yeast and rice or cut it into small pieces, put them into a bag and infuse them in spirits.

Actions:

> Strengthens the muscles, tendons and bones, relieves flaccid-

ity and arthralgia and lingering disease and restores *qi*.

Administration and Dosage:

    Oral administration.

Source:

    A Handbook of Family Dietetic Therapy, 1982, p. 512.

13. Wine of Lard

Ingredients:

    Lard and ginger juice 300 grams each.

Pharmaceutical Process:

    Decoct them together, mix their extract with 1,500 grams of millet wine and decoct the mixture.

Actions:

    Moistens the lungs and nourishes the muscles and tendons.

Indications:

    Overstrain, pains of the nails and inability to stand for long induced by exhaustion of the fluids of the limbs.

Administration and Dosage:

    50ml doses, twice per day.

Source:

    Collection of Prescriptions with Annotations

Section Twenty-one   Diabetes

The symptoms of diabetes are polydipsia, polyphagia, polyuria, magersucht and cloudy and sweet urine.

1. Spirit of Bayberry

Ingredients:

    Fruit of bayberry, spirits *q. s.*

Pharmaceutica Process:

Let the fresh fruit infuse airtight in the spirit for a long time.

Actions:

Quenches thirst, promotes digestion, dredges the stomach and the intestines and the five viscera, dispels dysphoria, stops vomiting and relieves diarrhea.

Administration and Dosage:

Oral administration.

Source:

A Handbook of Family Dietetic Therapy, 1982, p. 93.

2. Wine of Silkworm Chrysalises

Ingredients:

Silkworm chrysalises 30 grams, a cup of millet wine, a cup of water.

Pharmaceutical Process:

Boil them down to one cup of extract.

Indications:

Diabetes, dysphoria.

Administration and Dosage:

Take it at one draught.

Source:

Chinese Medicated Dietetics, 1985, p. 337.

3. Fermented Mulberry Fruit and Rice

Ingredients:

Fresh mulberry fruit 1,000 grams, glutinous rice 500 grams.

Pharmaceutical Process:

Wash the fruit clean, pound it to obtain the juice (or decoct 300 grams of dry mulberry fruit and remove the dregs and obtain the juice) and decoct the juice with the rice till they get thick. Mix them with some distiller's yeast when they cool down to let them ferment.

Actions:

Nourishes the blood, tonifies the kidneys, improves hearing and eyesight.

Indications:

Deficiency of *yin* of the liver and the kidneys, diabetes, constipation, tinnitus and eye failure, etc.

Administration and Dosage:

Oral administration with meals.

Source:

Chinese Medicated Dietetics, 1985, p. 208.

Section Twenty-two   Neurosism

Neurosism is common to mental workers or workers in specialized professions. It is a functional cerebral disturbance and is caused by the imbalance of cerebral excitement and inhibitory process and the disturbance of regular neural activities. Its clinical symptoms mainly include acratia, excitability, absent-mindedness, hypomnesis, dizziness, headache, insomnia and palpitation.

1. Spirit of Red Sage

Ingredients:

Red sage root 300 grams, spirits (containing 50% alcohol) *q. s.* (or millet wine).

Pharmaceutical Process:

Mince the herb, let it infuse in spirits for 15 days, filtrate the infusion and press the dregs to obtain extract. Mix it with the filtrate, add spirits to increase the quantity of the mixture to 1,000 ml, filtrate the mixture and again increase the quantity of the filtrate to 1,000ml by adding spirits.

Actions:

Nourishes the blood and promotes blood circulation.

Indication:

Neurosism.

Administration and Dosage:

Oral administration, 10ml doses, 3 times per day.

Storage:

Keep it airtight.

Sources:

1. Institute of Chinese Medicine of Shanxi Province *Pharmaceutical Techniques of Chinese Medicine*, 1982, p. 215.

2. *Common Preparations of Medicine*, ed. College of Pharmacy of Shenyang.

2. Tranquilization Spirit

Ingredients:

Siberian solomonseal rhizome 250 grams, steam of desertliving cistanche 250 grams, spirits containing 50% alcohol *q. s.*

Pharmaceutical Process:

Pound the herbs into samll pieces and make 1,000ml of medicinal spirits by means of extraction by infusion in cold spirit.

Indications:

Insomnia and amnesia.

Administration and Dosage:

Oral administration, 5—10ml doses, 3 times per day.

Source:

Department of Pharmaey of Beijing Medical College, *Pharmacy and Preparations with Annotation*, Fascicle 3, Vol, 2, 1976.

3. Spirit of Fleece-Flower Root

Ingredients:

Prepared fleece-flower root and rhizome of rehmannia 150 grams each; spirits 10,000 grams.

Pharmaceutical Process:

Wash the fleece-flower root clean, soak it till it gets soft and cut it into 1cm cubes. Cut the washed rehmannia into thin slices, airdry them, put the cubes and slices into a jar, then add the spirits slowly and mix them well. Seal up the jar and let the herbs infuse for 10—15 days, stirring them once every three days, and finally filtrate the infusion.

Actions:

Nourishes the liver and the kidneys, replenishes vital essence and blood and tonifies *yin*. Rehmannia can reduce the heat of spirits. It also builds up health and prolongs life.

Indications:

Dizziness, acratia, magersucht, lumbago, spermatorrhea, amnesia and premature poliosis induced by the deficiency of the liver and the kidneys, neurosis and copos.

Source:

Chinese Medicated Dietetics, 1985, p. 196.

4. Wine of Glossy Privet

Ingredients:

Glossy privet fruit 60 grams, yellow millet wine 500 grams.

Pharmaceutical Process:

Let the fruit infuse in the wine for 7 days.

Indication:

neurosism.

Administration and Dosage:

10ml doses, once or twice per day.

Source:

Chinese Medicated Dietetics, 1985, p. 214.

5. Spirit of Lucid Ganoderma

Ingredients:

Fruitification of lucid ganoderma 30 grams, spirits 500 grams.

Pharmaceutical Process:

Let the fungus infuse in the spirits for 7 days.

Indications:

Neurosism.

Administration and Dosage:

20—30ml doses, 2—3 times per day.

Source:

Chinese Medicated Dietetics

Remarks:

It can treat coronary disease with the addition of pseudo-ginseng and red sage root.

6. Spirit of Longan Pulp

Ingredionts:

Longan pulp 30 grams, spirits 500 grams.

Pharmaceutical Process:

Let the pulp infuse in the spirit for 1—3 months.

Actions:

Strengthens the stomach and the spleen and is refreshing.

Administration and Dosage:

10ml doses, 2—3 times per day.

Source:

Chinese Medicated Dietetics, 1985, p. 207.

Remarks:

50,000 grams of longan pulp can be made into 15,000 grams of 75% proof spirits.

A Handbook of Family Dietetic Therapy, 1892, p. 105.

7. Spirlt of Chinese Magnoliavine (I)

Ingredients:

Fruit of Chinese magnoliavine 30 grams, spirits 500 grams.

Pharmaceutical Process:

Let the fruit infuse in the spirits for 7 days.

Indications:

Acratia, debilitation, palpitation and insomnia.

Administration and Dosage:

10—20ml doses, once or twice per day.

Source:

Chinses Medicated Dietetics, 1985, P. 197.

8. Spirit of Chinese Magnoliavine (II)

Ingredients:

Fruit of Chinese magnoliavine 150 grams, spirits 500 grams.

Pharmaceutical Process:

Parch the fruit till it is done, grind it into small pieces and let them soak in the spirit for 1 month.

Actions:

Relieves mental distress.

Indication:

Insomnia.

Administration and Dosage:

15 gram doses, 3 times per day.

Source:

Medicinal Nourishment and Dietetic Nourishment···?

9. Spirit of Tranquilization

Ingredients:

Longan pulp 500 grams, osmanthus flowers 120 grams, sugar 240 grams, spirits 5,000 grams.

Pharmaceutical Process:

Let the pulp, flowers and sugar soak in the spirit for half a month.

Indications:

Insomnia and amensia.

Administration and Dosage:

Oral administration.

Source:

Strengthening Primordial Qi to Prolong Life

10. Spirit of Chinese Wolfberry and Longan

Ingredients:

Fruit of Chinese wolfberry 150 grams, longan pulp 200 grams, spirits 1,000 grams.

Pharmaceutical Process:

Let the fruit and pulp soak in the spirit for 14 days.

Actions:

Nourishes the heart and the kidneys, strengthens the mind and relieves mental distress.

164

Indications:

Vertigo, insomnia and dreaminess.

Administration and Dosage:

20ml doses, twice per day.

Source:

Medicinal Standards of Shanghai

11. Wine of *Codonopsis Pilosula* and Chinese Wolfberry

Ingredients:

Root of *Codonopsis pilosula* and fruit of Chinese wolfberry 15 grams each; millet wine 500 grams.

Pharmaceutical Process:

Let the root and fruit soak in the wine for 7 days.

Indications:

Neurosism, palpitation, amensia, insomnia and dreaminess.

Administration and Dosage:

15ml doses, twice per day in the morning and the evening.

Source:

Medicinal Nourishment and Dietetic Nourishment

12. Spirit of Chinese Angelica and Longan

Ingredients:

Rhizome of Chinese angelica 30 grams, longan pulp 240 grams.

Pharmaceutical Process:

Let the ingredients soak in 1,000 grams of spirits.

Indications:

Insomnia, amensia and senile debilitation.

Administration and Dosage:

20ml doses, twice per day.

Source:

3 Methods of Dietetic Nourishment

13. Raisin Wine

Ingredient:

raisins 500 grams.

Pharmaceutical Process:

Grind the raisins and let them infuse in 1,000 grams of millet wine for half a month.

Action:

Warms the kidneys.

Indications:

Palpitation, hyperhidrosis, edema, soreness in the waist and difficulty in urination.

Administration and Dosage:

30ml doses, twice per day.

Source:

Peaceful Holy Benevolent Prescriptions

14. Spirit of Lucid Ganoderma

Ingredients:

Fruitication of lucid ganoderma 25 grams, spirits 500 ml.

Pharmaceutical Process:

Let the fungus infuse in the spirit for 7 days.

Indication:

Neurosism.

Administration and Doage:

25ml doses, once per day.

Source:

1,100 Folk Prescriptions of Dietetic Therapy, 1992, p. 120.

Section Twenty-three   Climacteric Syndrome

Climacterium is an inevitable stage of the physiological development of men and women. The disturbance of endocrine function induces a lot of clinical syndromes, including vegetative nerve functional disturbance, which is manifested more remarkably in women.

1. Spirit of Eucommia and Ginseng

Ingredients:

Eucommia bark 30 grams, a ginseng root, spirits.

Pharmaceutical Process:

Wash the bark clean and let it infuse with the ginseng root in the spirits for 10—15 days.

Indication:

Climacterium of women.

Administration and Dosage:

50ml doses, twice per day.

Source:

1,100 *Folk Prescriptions of Dietetic Therapy*, 1992, p. 234.

2. Spirit of Curculigo and Epimedium

Ingredients:

Rhizome of curculigo and epimedium 15 grams each; morinda root 12 grams, Sichuan aborvitae seed and each, rhizome of wind —weed 6 grams, Chinese angelica root 10 grams spirits 1,000 grams.

Pharmaceutical Process:

Let the herbs infuse in the spirits for 21 days, filtrate the infusion, add some warm water to the dregs and decoct them for 20 minutes. Mix the decoction with the filtrate when it cools down and pour the mixture into another container for future use.

Actions:

Warms and nourishes the kidney-*yang*.

Indication:

Climacterium.

Administration and Dosage:

30 gram doses, twice per day.

Source:

Encyclopedia of Daily Life, Issue 7, 1986, p. 32.

Section Twenty-four   Consumptive Diseases

Consumptive diseases are induced by various factors and include the deficiency of the viscera, *qi*, blood, *yin* and *yang*, which brings about many chronic and debilitating illnesses.

1. Tonic Spirit

Ingredients:

Ginseng root (without head) 100 grams, pilose antler (hairless) and longan pulp 50 grams each; sliced Sichuan aconite root 100 grams, dried orange peel 150 grams, cibot rhizome (without villus, fruit of Chinese wolfberry and psoralea fruit (prepared in salt water) 200 grams each; Siberian solomonseal rhizome (stir-fried in spirit) 100 grams, cherokee rosehip (without villus), seed of Chinese chives 200 grams, *Epimedium brevicornum E. koreanum* (prepared in sheep oil) 200 grams, Chinese caterpillar fungus 100 grams, achyranthes root (without head) 200 grams, lucid ganoderma frutification 200 grams, Chinese angelica root 100 grams, finger citron fruit 100 grams, donkey kidney 100 grams,

168

50 sparrow heads (about 50 grams), brown sugar 3,000 grams, rice fermented with red yeast 400 grams, honey 5,000 grams.

Pharmaceutical Process:

Clean and prepare the ingredients, put them into a clean container and put the container into a reflux tank. Add 25,000 grams of 90% proof spirits; half an hour after boiling, add a further 15,000 grams of the same spirits and 10,000 grams more after another half an hour. Also add the rice fermented with red yeast at the same intervals of half an hour. Draw off each infusion respectively, press the dregs to obtain extract, then mix it with the three infusions. Keep the mixture static for a month, filtrate it and pack it separately in 500-gram bottles.

The medicated spirit is an orange-red liquid, which smells fragrant and tastes pungent and slightly bitter. Each 500-gram bottle has a tolerance of less than 1%. The spirit should be 70—78% proof.

Actions:

Nourishes blood and *qi* and strengthens the kidney-*yang*.

Indications:

General debilitation, lassitude, soreness and weakness of the waist and legs, impotence, deficiency of the kidneys, spermatorrhea, premature ejaculation and leukorrhea.

Administration and Dosage:

Oral administration, 15—25 gram doses, 2—3 times per day.

Caution:

Those with deficiency of *yin* and hyperactivity of *yang* must not take it.

Source:

Norms of Preparations of Chinese Medicine of Beijing, ed.
Bureau of Public Health of Beijing, 1974, p. 88.

2. Spirit of Lamb

Pharmaceutical Process:

Make spirit with a lamb.

Actions:

Highly tonic.

Source:

Essentials of Diet, vol. 3, *Spirit*

Ingredient:

Mutton 2,500 grams.

Pharmaceutical Process:

Steam the mutton till it is well-done, let it infuse in spirit for a night, then add 7 pears, pound them, add distiller's yeast and rice and make wine from them.

Actions:

Replenishes vital essence, strengthens the spleen and the stomach and nourishes the kidneys.

Source:

Compendium of Materia Medica.

3. Spirlt of *Poria Cocos*

Ingredients:

Sclerotium of *Poria cocos*.

Pharmaceutical Process:

Make medicated spirit with it.

Indication:

Consumptive disease.

Actions:

Strengthens the muscles, tendons and bones and prolongs life.
Source:

Essentials of Diet, vol. 3, Spirit.
or
Ingredients:

Sclerotium of *Poria cocos* 60 grams, spirits 500ml.
Pharmaceutical Process:

Infuse the sclerotium in the spirits, seal up the bottle and let the herb infuse for 7 days, shaking the bottle frequently.
Action:

Strengthens the spleen, stomach, muscles, tendons and bones.
Indications:

Numbness of the muscles and magersucht induced by deficiency of the spleen and stomach and malnutrition of the limbs.
Administration and Dosage:

Oral administration, 10ml dose per day before sleep or with a meal.

4. Spirit of Ginseng and Pilose Antler
Ingredients:

Red ginseng, pilose antler, morinda root, psoralea fruit, dodder seed, fruit of Chinese wolfberry, actinolite, cassia bark, aconite root, prepared rhizome of rehmannia, fruit of amomum, fossil of *Cyrtiospirifer sinensis*, root bark of Chinese wolfberry, eucommia bark, licorice root, buds of *Syzygium aromaticum Merr.*, dried sparrows, *Epimedium brevicornum E. Koreanum*, seahorse, lucid asparagus root, stem of *Cynomorium songaricum*, achyranthes root, halite, sulphur, seed of Chinses chives, donkey penis, dog penis, marten penis, hedgehog skin, desertliving cistanche, sorghum spirit, sugar.

Actions:

Replenishes vital essence and blood, nourishes the bones and brain and tonifies *yin* and *yang*.

Indications:

Lassitude, lumbago and backache, impotence, spermatorrhea, premature ejeculation; cold in the womb and sterility induced by deficiency of *yang* with the following symptoms: vertigo, tinnitus, insomnia, amensia, weakness of the limbs and knees, lack of appetite, lassitude, deep and floating pulse, pale tongue with white fur, deficiency of the kidney-*qi* and vital essence, astysia, weak erection, soreness and weakness of the waist, cold limbs, pale face, seminal emission, general debilitation, trance, menoxenia, scanty and pale menstruation, cold in the lower part of the abdomen, delayed menstruation, soreness of the waist, vague pain in the abdomen, slow and heavy pulse and pale tongue with thin and white fur during menstruation.

Administration and Dosage:

Oral administration, 10-15ml doses, 3 times per day.

Source:

Medicinal Standards of Liaojing Province (1976) in *Basic Preparations of Chinese Medicine*, vol. 1 1986, p. 236.

5. Spirit of Ginseng

Ingredients:

Ginseng 30 grams, spirits 500ml.

Pharmaceutical Process:

Put the ginseng into a gauze bag, decoct it in the spirits, seal up the bag and let the ginseng infuse in the spirit for 7 days.

Action:

Replenishes the middle-*jiao* and *qi*.

Indications:

Deficiency of *qi*, intolerance of cold, short breath induced by little work, spontaneous perspiration, acratia and loss of lustre and color of the face.

Administration and Dosage:

10ml doses, twice per day.

Source:

Compendium of Materia Medica.

6. Spirit of Siberian Solomonseal

Ingredients:

Rhizome of Siberian solomonseal and rhizome of Chinese a-tractylodes 200 grams each, root bark of Chinese wolfberry biota tops 2,500 grams, rhizome of asparagus 1,500 grams, distiller's yeast 5,000 grams, glutinous rice 50,000 grams.

Pharmaceutical Process:

Decoct the herbs, obtain 50,000 grams of extract from the decoction and make spirit from it with the yeast and rice; or let one-tenth of each of the herbs infuse airtight in 5,000 grams of spirit for 7 days, shaking the container frequently.

Actions:

Strengthens the spleen and nourishes the kidneys.

Indications:

Edema induced by deficiency of *yin* and dryness of the blood, dry and itchy skin, dysphoria, insomnia and withered beard and hair and premature greying.

Administration and Dosage:

10ml with meals.

Source:

Compendium of Materia Medica.

7. Spirit of Ginseng and Chinese Wolfberry

Ingredients:

Ginseng 200 grams, fruit of Chinese wolfberry 3,500 grams, prepared rhizome of rehmannia 1,000 grams, rock candy 4,000 grams, spirits 100,000 grams.

Pharmaceutical Process:

Bake the ginseng over a slow fire till it gets soft, cut it into slices, remove the impurities from the wolfberry fruit, put them into a gauze bag and tie up the mouth. Heat the candy in water till it melts, boils and turns yellow and filtrate it with gauze while it is still hot. Then let the ginseng slices and wolfberry fruit infuse in the spirits in a sealed jar for 10-15 days, stirring them once a day. Filtrate the infusion to remove the settled dregs, add the candy, mix them well and keep the mixture static for some time. Finally, filtrate it to obtain clear extract.

Actions:

Nourishes *yin* and the blood, blackens beard and hair, strengthens the waist and knees, improves eyesight, removes the obstruction in the collaterals and channels to promote blood circulation, dispels heat and promotes the production of body fluids.

Indications:

Lack of appetite, acratia, spontaneous perspiration, dizzi-

174

ness, insomnia, lumbago, copos, anemia, malnutrition, neurosism and diabetes.

Source:

Tongrentang of Chengdu, *Chinese Medicated Dietetics*, 1985, p. 184.

8. Spirit of Chinese Caterpillar Fungus

Ingredients:

Chinese caterpillar fungus 15—30 grams, spirits 500 grams.

Pharmaceutical Process:

Let the fungus infuse in the spirit for 7 days.

Indications:

Copos, lack of appetite, acratia and insomnia.

Administration and Dosage:

10-20ml doses, 2—3 times per day.

Source:

Chinese Medicated Dietetics, 1985, p. 228.

9. Spirit of Longan Pulp

Ingredients:

Longan pulp 200 grams, 60% proof spirits 400ml.

Pharmaceutical Process:

Let the pulp infuse airtight in the spirits for half a month.

Indications:

Consumptive diseases, debilitation, palpitation and insomnia.

Administration and Dosage:

10-20ml doses, twice per day.

Source:

Chinese Dietetic Therapeutics, p. 369.

10. Spirit of Snakes

Ingredients:

One or two live black-tail snakes or pallas-pit vipers, spirits.

Pharmaceutical Process:

Let the snakes infuse in the spirit for 10—15 days.

Indications:

Deuteropathic or postpartum anemia.

Administration and Dosage:

5-10ml doses, twice per day.

Source:

Chinese Dietetic Therapeutics, p. 371.

11. Spirlt of Ginseng and Longan

Ingredients:

Sun cured ginseng and candied ginseng 50 grams each; longan pulp 200 grams, rhizome of polygonatum 80 grams, granular sugar 1,600 grams, 52% proof spirits 22,400 grams.

Pharmaceutical Process:

Mince the herbs, let them infuse in 4,800 grams of the spirits for 14 days and remove the dregs. Heat the sugar in water to melt it, filtrate it, mix it with the medicinal spirits and the remaining spirits, keep the mixture static for 14 days and finally filtrate it.

Indications:

Deficiency of *qi* and the blood, lassitude and acratia, lack of appetite and insomnia.

Administration and Dosage:

20ml doses, twice per day.

Source:

12. Spirit of Deer Blood

Ingredient:

Deer blood.

Pharmaceutical Process:

Mix the blood drawn from the carotid of a deer and spirits to make spirit of deer blood 60% proof.

Indications:

Thrombocytopenia, leukopenia, aplastic anemia and hematopathy induced by chronic benzolism.

Administration and Dosage:

10ml doses, 3 times per day.

Source:

A Dictionary of Chinese Medicine

13. Wine of Strawberries

Ingredients:

Fresh strawberries.

Pharmaceutical Process:

Wash them clean, wrap them in gauze, squeeze out the juice and mix it with millet wine of equal quantity.

Indications:

Copos, magersucht and malnutrition.

Administration and Dosage:

30 gram doses, twice per day.

Source:

Medicinal Fruit

14. Spirit of Slender Acanthopanax

Ingredients:

Rhizome of slender acanthopanax 60 grams, spirits 1,000 grams.

Pharmaceutical Process:

Let the herb infuse in the spirit for half a month.

Actions:

Nourishes *qi* and strengthens the *spleen*.

Indications:

Deficiency of *qi*, acratia, lack of appetite and loose stools.

Administration and Dosage:

15ml doses, twice per day.

Source:

Proved Prescriptions

15. Wine of *Poria Cocos*

Ingredients:

Poria cocos 60 grams, millet wine 1,000 grams.

Pharmaceutical Process:

Let the ground herb infuse in the wine for 7 days.

Indications:

Deuteropathic debility, general acratia, chronic loose stool and chronic gastritis.

Administration and Dosage:

20ml doses, twice per day.

Source:

Compendium of Materia Medica

16. *Zhougong* Spirit

Ingredients:

Sclerotium of *Poria cocos* with host wood 90 grams, root of astragalus (stir-fried in a liquid) 60 grams; rhizome of rehmannia, prepared rhizome of rehmannia and Chinese angelica root 36 grams each; root of *Codonopsis Pilosula*, rhizome of large-headed atractylodes, tuber of dwarf lilyturf, fruit of dogwood, fruit of Chinese wolfberry, dried orange peel, rhizome of Ligusticum Chuanxiong, ledebouriella root and glue of freshwater turtle shell 30 grams each; fruit of schisandra and noterpterygium root 24 grams each; cassia bark 18 grams, spirits.

Pharmaceutical Process:

Let the herbs and glue infuse in the spirits for 21 days.

Actions:

Nourishes the blood and *qi* and removes the obstruction in the channels and collaterals to promote blood circulation.

Indications:

Consumptive diseases and hemiparalysis.

Administration and Dosage:

Oral administration in the morning and the evening.

Source:

Practical Preparations of Chinese Medicine in *Pharmacopoeia of Preparations of Chinese Medicine*, 1991, p. 882.

17. Tonic Spirit

Ingredients:

Root of *Codonopsis pilosula* and astragalus root 10 grams each; *Poria cocos* 12 grams, licorice root (stir-fried in a liquid) 6 grams, rhizome of large-headed atractylodes 10 grams, Chinese angelica root 10 grams, rhizome of Ligusticum Chuanxiong 3 grams, prepared rhizome of rehmannia, root of herbaceous peony 10 grams, cassia bark 3 grams, spirits 1,000 grams.

Pharmaceutical Process:

Let the herbs infuse in the spirits for 21 days, filtrate the infusion and decoct the dregs in some water for 20 minutes after boiling; filtrate the decoction when it cools down, mix the filtrates and pour the mixture into another container for future use.

Indications:

Deficiency of the blood and *qi*, consumptive disease and traumatic injury.

Administration and Dosage:

30 grams doses, twice per day.

Source:

Encyclopedia of Life, Issue 7, 1986, p. 32.

18. Tonic Spirit of Ginseng

Ingredients:

Ginseng and astragalus root 15 grams each, rhizome of large-headed atractylodes 10 grams, *Poria cocos* 10 grams, dried orange peel 3 grams, cassia bark 2 grams, Chinese angelica root 6 grams, licorice root stir-fried in a liquid 5 grams, spirits 1,000 grams.

Pharmaceutical Process:

Let the herbs infuse in the spirit for 21 days, filtrate them, add some warm water to the dregs and boil them for 20 minutes. When the decoction cools down, mix it and the filtrate and pour the mixture into a container.

Indications:

Deficiency of *qi* and blood, consumptive diseases and traumatic injury.

Administration and Dosage:

Oral administration, 30 gram doses, twice per day.

Source:

Encyclopedia of Life, Issue 7, 1986, p. 32.

19. Spirit of Rehmannia

Ingredients:

Prepared rhizome of rehmannia 250 grams, resinous wood of *Aquitaria sinensis* and fruit of Chinese wolfberry 200 grams each, sorghum spirit 2,500 grams.

Pharmaceutical Process:

Dry the rehmannia in sunlight, bake the wolfberry fruit and let the resinous wood infuse in the spirit for 10 days.

Actions:

Nourishes the liver and the kidneys and replenishes vital essence and blood.

Indications:

Deficiency of the liver, the kidneys, vital essence and blood, dizziness and soreness and weakness of the waist and knees.

Administration and Dosage:

10ml. before sleep.

Source:

Complete Works of Zhang Jingyue

20. Spirit of Ginseng

Ingredients:

Ginseng, prepared rhizome of rehmannia and Schisandra fruit **10** grams; tuber of dwarf lilyturf, Chinese angelica root and *Epimedium brevicornum E. Koreanum* (prepared with sheep oil) **15** grams each; spirits **500** grams.

Pharmaceutical Process:

Let the herbs infuse in the spirit.

Actions:

Nourishes *qi* and blood and warms and tonifies the liver and the kidneys.

Indications:

Deficiency of *qi* and blood, spermatorrhea, impotence (with symptoms of lack of appetite, loose stool, pallor, acratia, dizziness, spermatorrhea, impotence and weakness of the waist and knees), amensia, neurosism and sexual disorders.

Administration and Dosage:

Oral administration, 5-10ml doses, 2—3 times per day.

Source:

Practical Preparations of Chinese Medicine, 1991, p. 826.

Section Twenty-five Prolonging Life

Everybody wishes for health and longevity. As their living standard is raised, people desire a life of high quality and good health is the foundation for the attainment of this goal. Medicinal spirits can not only cure diseases, but also prevent them and build up health to prolong one's life.

1. Spirit for Longevity

Ingredients:

Siberian solomonseal rhizome and rhizome of asparagus 30 grams each; pine leaves 15 grams, fruit of Chinese wolfberry 20 grams, rhizome of Chinese atractylodes 12 grams, spirits 1,000 grams.

Pharmaceutical Process:

Cut the Siberian solomonseal rhizome, rhizome of asparagus and rhizome of Chinese atractylodes into 0.8 cm cubes, cut the

182

pine leaves into short segments and put them with the wolfberry fruit into a bottle. Add the spirits and let the herbs infuse for about 10-12 days.

Actions:

Nourishes the middle-*jiao*, replenishes vital essence and blood, tonifies the lungs and the kidneys, improves eyesight, prevents cold, builds up health and prolongs life.

Indications:

Rheumatism, general debilitation, lack of appetite, acratia and dizziness.

Source:

Zhongcangjing

2. Spirit of Ginseng

Ingredients:

Ginseng 10-20 grams, spirits 500 grams.

Pharmaceutical Process:

Let the ginseng infuse in the spirits for 7 days.

Actions:

Restores *qi*, builds up health and slows down senility.

Administration and Dosage:

5-10ml doses, twice per day.

Source:

Chinese Medicated Dietetics, 1985, p. 194.

3. Spirit of Chinese Angelica and Longan

Ingredients:

Chinese angelica root, longan pulp.

Pharmaceutical Process:

Let them infuse in good spirit.

Actions:

Nourishes blood and improves complexion.

Administration and Dosage:

A little per day.

Source:

A Handbook of Family Dietetic Therapy, 1982, p. 509.

4. Spirit of Chinese Wolfberry

Ingedients:

Fruit of Chinese wolfberry 30-60 grams, spirits 500 grams.

Pharmaceutical Process:

Let the fruit infuse in the spirit for 7 days.

Actions:

Nourishes *yin* and blood, replenishes vital essence, improves eyesight, builds up health and prolongs life.

Indications:

Dizziness, blurred vision, acratia of the waist and the knees, impotence.

Administration and Dosage:

5-15ml doses, 2—3 times per day.

Source:

Chinese Medicated Dietetics, 1985, p. 206.

5. Wine of Asparagus

Ingredients:

Rhizome of asparagus 30 grams, glutinous rice 500 grams.

Pharmaceutical Process:

Decoct the asparagus, make wine from the extract of the decoction, distiller's yeast and the rice.

Actions:

Nourishes *yin*, dispels heat, moistens the lungs and promotes the production of body fluids and builds up health.

Administration and Dosage:

10-30ml each time.

Source:

Chinese Medicated Dietetics, 1985, p. 210.

6. Spirit of Dodder and Schisandra

Ingredients:

Dodder seed and fruit of schisandra 30 grams each; spirits 500 grams.

Pharmaceutical Process:

Let the herbs infuse in the spirit for 7 days.

Actions:

Builds up health and prolongs life.

Indications:

Lumbago, dizziness and spermatorrhea induced by the deficiency of the liver and the kidneys.

Administration and Dosage:

20-30ml doses, 2—3 times per day.

Source:

Chinese Medicated Dietetics, 1985, p. 226.

7. Spirit of Fleece-Flower and Siberian Solomonseal

Ingredients:

Fleece-flower root and Siberian solomonseal rhizome 30 grams each; spirits 500 grams.

Pharmaceutical Process:

Wash the herbs clean, cut them into small slices, wrap them in gauze, tie up the gauze and let the herbs infuse in the spirits for 15 days.

Actions:

Blackens hair and prolongs life.

Administration and Dosage:

Once per day before sleep, 15-30ml.

Source:

1,100 *Folk Prescriptions of Dietetic Therapy*, 1992, p. 139.

8. Spirlt of Fleece-Flower Roots

Ingredients:

Red and white fleece-flower roots 500 grams each, rhizome of rehmannia and ginger juice 120 grams each; stoned fruit of jujube, walnut kernels and lotus seed 90 grams each; Chinese angelica rhizome and fruit of Chinese wolfberry 60 grams each; tuber of dwarf lilyturf 30 grams and millet wine 7,500 grams.

Pharmaceutical Process:

Let the herbs and fruits infuse in the wine for half a month, remove the dregs and add 90 grams of honey.

Actions:

Blackens beard and hair and prolongs life.

Administration:

3 cups per day.

Source:

Nourishing Primordial Qi to Prolong Life.

Section Twenty-six   Tentanus

Tetanus is an acute infectious disease induced by bacillus tetani and its clinical symptoms are lockjaw, clonic spasm, rigidity and opisthotonus, etc.

1. Spirit of Hemp

Ingredients:

Hemp skin 120 grams.

Pharmaceutical Process:

Grill it over charcoal fire till its crust chares but its original properties are retained. Grind it into fine powder, divide the powder into 4 doses and add yellow millet wine or spirits *q. s.* to each dose according to each patient's capacity for spirits. Drink it with boiled water.

Indication:

Tetanus.

Administration and Dosage:

1 dose 2—3 times per day. After taking a dose, the patient should be covered with a quilt to induce diaphoresis.

Source:

The People's Hospital of Shuyang County, Jiangsu Province, *Selection of the Materials of the National Exhibition of Chinese Medicinal Herbs and New Therapy*, 1972, p. 286.

2. Spirit of Cottonseed

Ingredients:

Cottonseed 90 grams, small black soybeans 45 grams, scallion stalks (with roots and without leaves) 500 grams, spirits 75 grams.

Pharmaceutical Process:

Parch the cottonseed till it turns dark reddish purple, grind it and sift it to remove the shells. Decoct the scallion stalks in 800-1,000ml of water. Parch the soybeans in a big iron pan till 90% of them get crisp, remove the pan from the fire, add the warm spirits and filtrate the mixture. Mix the dark reddish purple filtrate and the cottonseed powder, add some scallion soup and stir them till the mixture looks like thin gruel.

Indication:

Tetanus.

Administration and Dosage:

Oral administration. After taking each dose, the patient should be covered with quilt to induce diaphoresis and the scallion soup should be taken for 1-2 days in succession.

Caution:

Do not eat fishy or cold food while taking the spirits.

Source:

Lixin County, Anhui Province, *Selection of the Materials of the National Exhibition of Chinese Medicinal Herbs and New Therapy*, 1972, p. 285.

Section Twenty-seven　Epilepsy

Epilepsy is a paroxysmal unconscious disease with symptoms of trance, sudden loss of consciousness, salivation, showing the whites of the eyes, convulsions and bleating or barking. The patient comes to when moved and returns to normal. The disease relapses irregularly.

1. Composite Rhubarb Spirit

Ingredients:

Root and rhizome of rhubarb 1,000 grams, ledebouriella root 500 grams.

Pharmaceutical Process:

Grind the herbs into small pieces, put them into a bottle, add

1,500 grams of spirits, let the herbs infuse for 14 days and filtrate the infusion.

Actions:

Promotes blood circulation and dispels cold.

Indication:

Epilepsy.

Administration and Dosage:

Oral administration, 10ml doses for adults, 3 times per day;
15ml doses for children 10—14 years old, 3 times per day; 5ml
doses for children under 10, once or twice per day.

Source:

Fuyang Medicine, Issue 2, 1972, p. 44.

2. Wine of Asparagus

Ingredients:

Rhizome of asparagus.

Pharmaceutical Process:

Decoct the rhizome in winter and make wine from its extract
with distiller's yeast and rice.

Actions:

Moistens the viscera and promotes blood circulation.

Indications:

Five kinds of impairments and seven kinds of impairments
and epilepsy.

Administration and Dosage:

Take it at short intervals.

Caution:

Do not get drunk or eat cold and raw food while taking the
spirits.

Source:

A Handbook of Family Dietetic Therapy, 1982, p. 511.

Section Twenty-eight   Scurvy

Also known as vitamin C deficiency, scurvy has the symptoms of red and swollen gums, subcutaneous hemorrhage, follicular keratosis, anaemia and fever.

1. Wine of Black Soybeans

Ingredients:

Black soybeans, haws and white sugar 120 grams each, yellow millet wine.

Pharmaceutical Process:

Pound the soybeans, haws and sugar together, add 3 cups of water, bring them to the boil and add the wine.

Indication:

Scurvy.

Administration and Dosage:

take it at one draught.

Source:

A handbook of Family Dietetic Therapy, 1982, p. 11.

Section Twenty-nine   Andropathy

This part mainly consists of prescriptions for male sexual disorders including asexuality, impotence, prospermia, spermatorrhea and enuresis, etc.

1. Spirit of *Epimedium Brevicornum*, *E. Koreanum*

Ingredients:

Epemedium brevicornum, *E. Koreanum*, spirits 500ml.

Pharmaceutical Process:

Put the herbs into a gauze bag and let them infuse airtight for 3 days.

Actions:

Nourishes the liver and kidneys; strengthens the muscles, tendons and bones.

Indications:

Deficiency of *yin* and *yang*, dysfuction of reproductive system due to insufficiency of the kidney-*yang*, impotence; sterility and numbness of the limbs in women.

Administration and Dosage:

10ml doses before sleep.

Source:

Compendium of Materia Medica.

2. Spirit of Seahorses

Ingredients:

Two sea horses, 500ml of spirits.

Pharmaceutical Process:

Let the seahorses infuse airtight in the spirit for 15 days, shaking the bottle frequently.

Actions:

Warms the kidneys and strengthens *yang*.

Indications:

Impotence and soreness and weakness of the waist and the knees induced by dysfunction of the reproductive system due to insufficiency of the kidney-*yang*.

Administration and Dosage:

10ml each time before sleep.

Source:

Food and Treatment

3. Spirit of Prawns

Ingredients:

Two live prawns, 250ml of spirits.

Pharmaceutical Process:

Wash the prawns clean, put them into a bottle, add the spirits and seal up the bottle. Let the prawns infuse in the spirits for a week, shaking the bottle every day.

Actions:

Nourishes the kidneys and strengthens *yang*.

Indications:

Hypogonadism and impotence.

Administration and Dosage:

Drink it according to individual capacity for spirits with or without meals. Cook the prawns, divide them into equal parts and eat them with meals after the spirits are drunk.

Source:

Supplement to the Compendium of Materia Medica

4. Spirit of *Epimedium Brevicornum*, *E. Koreanum*

Ingredients:

Leaves of *Epimedium Brevicornum*, *E. Koreanum qs.*, spirits *q. s.*

Pharmaceutical Process:

Wash the leaves clean, mince them and let them infuse in 900 grams of good spirit for 7 days. Filtrate the infusion, let the dregs infuse in a little spirits for a few days, then press them, filtrate them and mix the two filtrates (amounting to 900 grams in all and 66% proof).

Actions:

Nourishes the kidneys and strengthens *yang*.

Indications:

Deficiency of the kidney-*yang*, asexuality, impotence, premature ejaculation and spermatorrhea.

Administration and Dosage:

3—6 gram doses, 3 times per day, before meals and diluted with warm boiled water.

Source:

Practical and Proved Simple Recipes

5. Spirit of Desertliving Cistanche

Ingredients:

Fleshy stem of desertliving cistanche 50 grams, root of cyathula 40 grams; morinda root (parched till it turns yellow) and red peppers 30 grams each; stir-baked ginger, cassia bark, dodder seed, prepared aconite root and seed of round cardamom 20 grams each; psoralea fruit and fruit of papermulberry 25 grams each; cnidium fruit and rhizome of birthwood 15 grams each; pilose antler (without hair and stir-fried in a liquid to make it crisp) 10 grams, spirits 1,500ml.

Pharmaceutical Process:

Pound the herbs and antler, put them into a bag and put the bag into a clean container. Let the herbs and pilose infuse in the spirit for 5-7 days and remove the dregs.

Actions:

Nourishes the kidneys and the liver and strengthens the muscles, tendons and bones.

Indications:

Deficiency of the liver and the kidneys and asexuality, impotence, premature ejaculation, dribbling urination, cold and pains in the waist and knees induced by cold and deficiency of qi of the lower part of the body.

Administration and Dosage:

10-15ml warm doses, twice per day before breakfast and supper.

Source:

Proved Folk Prescriptions.

6. Spirit of Chrysanthemum Flowers

Ingredients:

Chrysanthemum flowers, fruit of Chinese wolfberry, morinda root and fleshy stem of desertliving cistanche 90 grams each; spirits 2,000ml.

Pharmaceutical Process:

Remove the heart of the morinda, pound it with the other herbs, put them into a cloth bag and put the bag into a clean container. Add the spirits and seal up the container. Add 1,500ml of boiled water 7 days later, remove the dregs and pack the extract.

Actions:

Regulates primordial qi, improves eyesight and builds up health.

Indications:

Asexuality, arthralgia and myalgia, weakness of the limbs induced by insufficiency of primordial qi and cold and deficiency of qi of the lower part of the body.

Administration and Dosage:

Oral administration, 10-20ml doses, before breakfast and supper.

Source:

Proved Folk Prescriptions

7. Spirit of Ants

Ingredients:

Ants (dried) 20 grams, spirits 500ml.

Pharmaceutical Process:

Let the dried ants infuse in the spirit for a month. Then remove the ants and filtrate the spirits.

Actions:

Nourishes the kidneys and replenishes *qi*, builds up health, lusters the face and slows down senility.

Indications:

Deficiency of the kidney-*qi*, asexuality, impotence, premature ejaculation, deuteropathic alopecia and aplastic anemia-PNH syndrome.

Administration and Dosage:

20ml per day in winter.

Source:

Food and Sexual Hygiene

8. Spirit of Magnetite

Ingredients:

Magnetite 1,500 grams, spirits 15,000ml.

Pharmaceutical Process:

Grind the magnetite into powder and let it infuse in the spirits for over 10 days.

Actions:

Nourishes *yin* and the kidneys.

Indications:

Deficiency of the liver-*yin* and the kidney-*yin*, asexuality, dizziness, soreness and weakness of the waist and knees, tinnitus, bad hearing, dysphoria with feverish sensation in the chest, palms and soles, reddish tongue and thready pulse.

Administration and Dosage:

150ml doses, 3 times in daytime and once at night.

Source:

Prescriptions for Emergencies

9. Spirit of Deer Penises

Ingredients:

Two deer penises, spirits or millet wine 1,000ml.

Pharmaceutical Process:

Wash the penises clean, let them soak in warm water till they get soft, remove the inner membranes and cut them into thin slices. Let them infuse in the spirits or wine for a month.

Action:

nourishes the kidney-*yang*.

Indications:

Impotence, prepature ejeculation, acratia and lassitude induced by deficiency of the kidney-*yang*.

Administration and Dosage:

10-15ml doses, twice per day.

Source:

Food and Sexual Hygiene.

10. Spirit of Ursine Seal's Penis and Testes

Ingredients:

Ursine seal's penis and testes, glutinous rice and distiller's yeast *q. s.*

Pharmaceutical Process:

Infuse the penis and testes in spirits, pound them into pulp and make wine from them with the rice and the yeast.

Actions:

Replenishes *yang* and vital essence, dispels cold and consolidates the bones.

Indications:

Deficiency of the kidneys, acratia, impotence, spermatorrhea, cold sperm, cold and pains in the waist and knees and flaccidity.

Administration and Dosage:

10-15ml doese, twice per day.

Source:

Compendium of Materia Medica

11. Spirit of Ginseng and Chinese Wolfberry

Ingredients:

Ginseng 10 grams, fruit of Chinese wolfberry 175 grams, prepared rhizome of rehmannia 50 grams, rock candy 200 grams, spirits 500 ml.

Pharmaceutical Process:

Cut the ginseng into slices, remove the impurities from the wolfberry fruit and put them and the rehmannia into a gauze bag. Melt the candy, filtrate it, put the filtrate and the bag into the spirits, seal up the container and let them infuse for 10-15 days.

Actions:

Replenishes primordial *qi*, calms the mind and arrests spontaneous emission.

Indications:

Consumptive disease, traumatic injury, impotence, lack of appetite, lassitude, lumbago, weakness of the limbs and listlessness.

Administration and Dosage:

Once per day.

Source:

Medicated Recipes of Tongrentang of Chengdu

12. Spirit of *Cynomorium Songaricum*

Ingredients:

Fleshy stem of *Cynomorium songaricum* 30 grams, spirits 500 ml.

Pharmaceutical Process:

Let the herb infuse in the spirit for 7 days, remove the dregs and pour the extract into a bottle.

Actions:

Nourishes vital essence, replenishes the blood and strengthens *yang* and the muscles and tendons.

Indications:

Deficiency of the kidneys, impotence, weakness of the waist and knees, spermatorrhea, premature ejeculation, insufficieucy of the blood and vital essence, lassitude and withered face.

Administration and Dosage:

15-20ml doses, twice per day.

Source:

Food and Sexual Hygiene

13. Spirit Strengthening *Yang*

Ingredients:

Papermulberry fruit (parched for a short while) 50 grams, pilose antler (without hair and stir—fried in a liquid to make it crisp); prepared aconite root, root of cyathula, morinda root, stem of *Dendrobium nobile Lindl.* and jujube fruit 30 grams each ; stir-baked ginger and cassia bark 15 grams each, spirits 1,000ml.

Pharmaceutical Process:

Pound the herbs and fruit, put them into a cloth bag and put the bag into a clean container. Add the spirits, seal up the container, let them infuse for 8 days and remove the dregs.

Actions:

Nourishes the kidneys, strengthens *yang*, the muscles, tendons and bones and warms the spleen and the stomach.

Indications:

Impotence, spermatorrhea, premature ejeculation, deficiency and cold of the spleen and the stomach, lack of appetite and withered face induced by deficiency of the kidney-*yang*.

Administration and Dosage:

10ml before breakfast and supper respectively while it is warm.

Source:

Proved Folk Prescriptions

14. Spirit of Morinda

Ingredients:

Morinda root and chrysanthemum flowers 60 grams each, prepared rhizome of rehmannia 45 grams, fruit of Chinese wolfberry and Sichuan peppers 30 grams each, prepared aconite root 20 grams, good spirits 1,500ml.

Pharmaceutical Process:

Let the pounded herbs infuse in the spirits in a clean and sealed bottle for 5 days and remove the dregs.

Actions:

Nourishes the kidneys and strengthens *yang*.

Indications:

Impotence, premature ejeculation, soreness and weakness of the waist and knees, cold limbs, aversion to cold and lumbago induced by longstanding deficiency of the kidney-*yang*.

Administration and Dosage:

10-20ml before breakfast and supper while it is warm.

Source:

Proved Folk Prescriptions

15. Spirit of Ginseng

Ingredients:

White ginseng 50 grams, spirits *q. s.*

Pharmaceutical Process:

Infuse the pounded ginseng with 500ml of 60% proof spirits in a sealed flask for half a month, shaking it several times per day. Drink it while replenishing it with spirits to keep the quantity at 500ml.

Actions:

Nourishes the heart and tonifies the spleen.

Indications:

Neurosism, insomnia, lassitude, palpitation, short breath and impotence.

Administration and Dosage:

10-30ml at supper daily.

Source:

Collection of Medicated Recipes

16. Spirit of Pilose Antler

Ingredients:

Pilose antler 3-6 grams, Chinese yam 30-60 grams, spirits 500 grams.

Pharmaceutical Process:

Let the antler and yam infuse in the spirits in a sealed bottle for 7 days.

Actions:

Replenishes the kidney-*yang* and reinforces the gall bladder.

Indications:

Premature ejaculation, asexuality, lumbago, weakness of the knees, lassitude, listlessness, cold and pain in the lower part of the abdomen, frequent micturition at night, dribbling urination, withered face, pale tongue with white fur and deep and weak pulse.

Administration and Dosage:

10ml before sleep daily.

source:

Compendium of Materia Medica

17. Spirit of Chinese Wolfberry

Ingredients:

Dried fruit of Chinese wolfberry 200 grams, 60% proof spirits 300ml.

Pharmaceutical Process:

Infuse the cleaned and minced fruit in the spirits in a sealed flask for 7 days, shaking it once or twice every day. Drink it while replenishing the bottle with spirits *q. s.*

Actions:

Nourishes the liver and reinforces the kidneys.

Indications:

Premature ejeculation, blurred vision, dizziness, tinnitus, weakness and soreness of the waist and knees, magersucht, reddish tongue with thin fur and thready pulse induced by deficiency of the kidneys.

Administration and Dosage:

10-20ml either at supper or before sleep.

Source:

Peaceful Benevolent Holy Prescriptions.

18. Spirit of Curculigo

Ingredient:

Rhizome of curculigo

Pharmaceutical Process:

Let the herb, steamed and sunned nine times, infuse in the spirits.

Actions:

Warms the kidneys, invigorates *yang* and dispels cold.

Indications:

Cold sperm, dysfunction of the reproductive system due to insufficiency of the kidney-*yang*, cold limbs, acratia, lassitude, dampness and and cold of pudendum, pale tongue with thin and white fur and slow and weak pulse (at the proximal position in particular).

Administration and Dosage:

Oral administration at any time.

Source:

Compendium of Materia Medica

19. Wine of Dog Meat

Ingredient:

Meat of a yellow dog.

Pharmaceutical Process:

Cook the meat till it is well-done and make wine from the meat, the gravy, distiller's yeast and rice.

Action:

Replenishes the kidney-*yang*.

Indications:

Cold and thin sperm, sterility, cold and pains in the waist and knees, weakness of the lower limbs, lassitude, listlessness, darkish complexion, pale tongue with white and thin fur and weak pulse.

Administration and Dosage:

Drink it frequently at any time.

Caution:

Those with deficiency of *yin* and without cold-pain should not take it since it is very hot in nature.

Source:

Compendium of Materia Medica

20. Spirit of Siberian Solomonseal

Ingrdients:

Rhizome of Siberian solomonseal, rhizome of large-headed a-tractylodes and rhizome of asparagus 1,500 grams each; pine-leaves 3,000 grams, fruit of Chinese wolfberry 2,500 grams.

Pharmaceutical Process:

Decoct the ingredients in 15,000ml of water for a day, remove the dregs and make spirits from the extract and distiller's yeast.

Actions:

Replenishes vital essence and nourishes the liver and the spleen.

Indications:

General debilitation, susceptibility to diseases, cold and thin sperm, senilitis, premature greying of hair and odontoseisis, withered face, lack of appetite, anorexia, fullness in the chest, hypochondrium, soreness and weakness of the waist and knees.

Administration and Dosage:

Oral administration.

Source:

A Supplement to the Essential Prescriptions

21. Refreshing Spirits

Ingredients:

Fruit of Chinese wolfberry 30 grams; prepared rhizome of rehmannia, red ginseng and *Epimedium brevicornum*, *E. koreanum* 15 grams each; flatstem milkvetch seed 25 grams, resinous wood of *Aquilaria sinesis* 5 grams, litchi seed 12 grams, parched polygala root, cloves 6 grams.

Pharmaceutical Process:

Remove the impurities of the ingredients, mince them and let them infuse in 1,000 grams of spirits and 52 grams of rock candy for a month.

Actions:

Replenishes the blood, invigorates the function of the brains, replenishes vital essence and strengthens *yang*.

Indications:

Deficiency of the kidney-*yang*, cold sperm, sterility, lassitude, amnesia, listlessness, slow reaction, soreness and weakness of the waist and knees, micturition, precipitant urination, pale tongue with white and moist fur and weak and deep pulse.

Administration and Dosage:

Oral administration, 20ml in the evening.

Source:

Collection of Clinical Experience of Gong Zhixian

22. Spirit of Morinda

Ingredients:

Morinda root 60 grams, prepared rhizome of rehmannia 45 grams, fruit of Chinese wolfberry 30 grams, prepared aconite root 20 grams, dried chrysanthemum flowers 60 grams, Sichuan peppers 30 grams, good qualit spirits 1,500ml.

Pharmaceutical Process:

Let the pounded herbs infuse in the spirits in a clean and sealed bottle for 5 days and then remove the dregs.

Actions:

Warms the kidneys, dispels cold and promotes the flow of *qi*.

Indications:

Intermittent testicular pain which worsens when it is cold, soreness and weakness of the waist and knees, cold limbs, pale face with white fur and deep and slow pulse.

Administration and Dosage:

10-20ml before meals while it is warm.

Source:

Proved Folk Prescriptions

23. Spirit of Prepared Rehmannia

Ingredients:

Prepared rhizome of rehmannia 250 grams, resinous wood of *Aquilaria sinensis* 3 grams, fruit of Chinese wolfberry 120 grams, spirits 300ml.

Pharmaceutical Process:

Let the herbs infuse in the spirits in a clean and sealed container for 5 days.

Actions:

Replenishes blood and vital essence, relieves pain.

Indications:

Slight testicular pain, dizziness, tinnitus, weakness and soreness of the waist and knees, magersucht, dysphoria with feverish sensation in the chest, palms and soles; night sweats, reddish tongue with scanty fur, thready pulse.

Administration and Dosage:

Once per day.

Source:

Food and Sexual Hygiene

24. Composite Spirit of Pinellia

Ingredients:

Dried tangerine peel 30 grams, tuber of pinellia 24 grams, dried vascular bundles of tangerine mesocarp 18 grams, spirits 250ml.

Pharmaceutical Process:

206

Let the pounded herbs infuse in the spirits in a sealed container for 7 days, shaking it several times evry day. Filtrate the infusion, add 500ml of water to the filtrate, boil them for a few minutes, then add 5 grams of potassium iodide when they cool down.

Actions:

Softens and resolves hard masses formed by the accumulation of phlegm or blood stasis and promotes blood circulation.

Indications:

Swollen and tender penis with hard lumps but without abnormal change of the skin, sallow face, white and thin fur on the tongue and thready pulse.

Administration and Dosage:

Oral administration, 2ml doses after breakfast and supper. Drink a lot of boiled water after taking the spirit.

Source:

Miraculous Prescriptions

25. Wine of Slender Acanthopanax

Ingredients:

Root bark of slender acanthopanax, Chinese angelica root and achyranthes root 60 grams each; glutinous rice 1,000 grams, sweet wine.

Pharmaceutical Process:

Wash the herbs, decoct them and make wine with the extract, rice, wine and distiller's yeast.

Actions:

Dispels cold and dampness, nourishes the liver and the kidneys.

Indications:

Scrotal prurigo, withered face, dry eyes, vertigo, tinnitus, weakness and soreness of the knees and waist, pale tongue and thready pulse.

Administration and Dosage:

Oral administration.

Source:

Compendium of Materia Medica

26. Composite Spirit

Ingredients:

Dried vascular bundles of tangerine mesocarp 18 grams, tuber of pinellia 24 grams, dried tangerine peel parched with white mustard seed and stir-baked pangolin scales 30 grams each.

Pharmaceutical Process:

Grind the ingredients into small pieces, let them infuse in 300 ml of spirit in a sealed container for 7 days and filtrate the infusion. Add 500ml of water to the dregs, let them infuse for 1 day, then filtrate the infusion and mix the filtrates. Boil the mixture for 2 minutes in an earthenware pot, add 5 grams of potassium iodide when it cools down Finally, pour it into a bottle when the potassium iodide dissolves.

Actions:

Softens and resolves hard masses formed by the accumulation of phlegm or blood stasis and promotes blood circulation.

Indications:

Swollen penis with hard lumps and slight pain, fullness in the chest and hypochondrium, dark tongue with slimy fur.

Administration and Dosage:

2ml doses, 3 times after meals per day.

Source:

Journal of chinese Medicine of Zhejiang

27. Spirit of *Rana Limnocharis Boie*

Ingredients:

Good spirits 2,500 grams, *Rana limnocharis Boie*, rhizome of glabrous greenbrier 500 grams.

Pharmaceutical Process:

Put the rhizome, frog and spirits into a bottle, seal it up, put it into a pot with water and decoct the ingredients for 1-2 hours. Drink the spirit the next day.

Actions:

Dispels heat, toxic material and dampness, relieves pain.

Indications:

Syphilitic skin lesions, arthralgia and myalgia.

Source:

Orthodox Manual of External Diseases

28. Wine of Lophatherum

Ingredient:

Dried aerial parts of lophatherum 250 grams.

Pharmaceutical Process:

Decoct the leaves and make wine from the extract, distiller's yeast and rice.

Actions:

Dispels heat and promotes diuresis.

Indications:

Dark urine, difficulty in urination, burning sensation during urination, vexation, thirst, vomiting, aphthae, reddish tongue tip and slow pulse.

Administration and Dosage:

Drink it slowly at any time.

Source:

Collection of Proved Prescriptions of Medicated Spirits

29. Spirit of Ginseng and Ursine Seal

Ingredients:

Ursine seal's penis and testes, ginseng 15 grams, Chinese yam 30 grams.

Pharmaceutical Process:

Cut the penis and testes infused in spirit into slices and let them infuse with the ginseng and yam in 1,000 grams of spirits for 7 days.

Indications:

Deficiency of the kidneys, impotence, lassitude and listlessness.

Administration and Dosage:

10ml doses, twice per day.

Source:

Chinese Medicated Dietetics, 1985, p. 218.

30. Spirit of Stink-Bugs

Ingredients:

Stink-bugs 30 grams, spirits 500 grams.

Pharmaceutical Process:

Let the bugs infuse in the spirit for 7 days.

Indications:

Deficiency of the kidneys and impotence.

Administration and Dosage:

10-20ml doses, twice per day.

Source:

Chinese Medicated Dietetics, 1985, p. 218.

31. Spirit of Morinda

Ingredients:

Morinda root and achyranthes root 30 grams each; spirits 500 grams.

Pharmaceutical Process:

Let the herbs infuse in the spirits for 7 days.

Indications:

Deficiency of the kidneys, impotence and weakness of the feet.

Administration and Dosage:

10-20ml doses, twice per day.

Source:

Chinese Medicated Dietetics, 1985, p. 221.

32. Spirit of Cekko Gecko

Ingredients:

two dried Cekko gecko bodies with their viscera removed, yellow millet wine 500 grams.

Pharmaceutical Process:

Remove the feet and scales of the lizards and let them infuse in the wine for 7 days.

Indications:

Deficiency of the kidneys, impotence and frequent micturition.

Administration and Dosage:

10-20ml doses, twice per day.

Source:

Chinese Medicated Dietetics, 1985, p. 229.

33. Spirit of *Saussurea Laniceps Hand.-Mazz.*

Ingredients:

Saussurea laniceps Hand.-Mazz. 30 grams, spirits 500 grams.

Pharmaceutical Process:

Let the herb infuse in the spirits for 7 days.

Indications:

Impotence and rheumatic arthralgia.

Administration and Dosage:

10ml doses, twice per day.

Source:

Chinese Medicated Dietetics, 1985, p. 230.

34. Spirit of Desertliving Cistanche

Ingredients:

Desertliving cistanche 30 grams, spirits 500 grams.

Pharmaceutical Process:

Let the herb infuse in the spirit for 7 days.

Indications:

Deficiency of the kidneys and impotence.

Administration and Dosage:

10ml doses, twice per day.

Source:

Chinese Medicated Dietetics, 1985, p. 225.

35. Wine of Sparrows

Ingredients:

3-5 sparrows, seed of *Cuscuta chinensis* and desertliving cistanche 15 grams each; millet wine 1,000 grams.

Pharmaceutical Process:

Slaughter and clean the sparrows. Infuse them and the herbs in the wine for 7 days.

Actions:

Strengthens *yang*, replenishes *qi* and vital essence and reduces urination.

Indications:

Impotence, premature ejaculation, soreness and weakness of the waist and knees and senile deficiency of *yang*.

Administration and Dosage:

Oral administration.

Soruce:

A Handbook of Family Dietetic Therapy, 1982, p. 210.

36. Wine of *Momordica Charantia L.*

Ingredient:

Seed of *Momordica charantia L.* 15 grams.

Pharmaceutical Process:

Parch the seed till it is done, grind it into powder and take it with yellow millet wine.

Indication:

Impotence.

Administration and Dosage:

3 times per day (10 days constitute a cource of treatment).

Source:

A Handbook of Family Dietetic Therapy, 1982, p. 55.

37. Composite Spirit of Rehmannia

Ingredients:

Prepared rhizome of rehmannia 250 grams , resinous wood of *Aquilaria sinensis* or sandalwood 3 grams, fruit of Chinese wolfberry, spirits 3,000 grams.

Pharmaceutical Process:

Let the herbs infuse in the spirit for over 10 days.

Indications:

Deficiency of essence and blood, pain and weakness of the waist, vertigo, asexuality, etc.

Administration and Dosage:

Oral administration.

Source:

Chinese Medicated Dietetics, 1985, p. 203.

38. Lotus Leaf Powder

Ingredient:

Lotus leaf 9 grams.

Pharmaceutical Process:

Grind the leaf into powder and take it with spirits.

Indication:

Spermatorrhea.

Administration and Dosage:

Take it at one draught.

Source:

A Handbook of Family Dietetic Therapy, 1982, p. 73.

39. Spirit of Curculigo

Ingredients:

Curculigo rhizome 30 grams, spirits 500 grams.

Pharmaceutical Process:

Let the rhizome infuse in the spirits for 7 days.

Indications:

Senile enuresis and frequent urination.

Administration and Dosage:

10-20ml doses, twice per day.

Source:

Chinese Medicated Dietetics, 1985, p. 223.

40. Silk Moth Powder

Ingredient:

Silk moth 6 grams (ground to powder).

Pharmaceutical Process:

Mix it with hot spirits.

Indications:

Stranguria complicated by hematuria, stranguria round the navel and in the abdomen and penis.

Administration and Dosage:

Take it in one draught.

Source:

Peaceful Holy Benevolent Prescriptions

41. Spirit of Flowers of Chinese Chives

Ingredients:

Resinous wood of *Aquilaria sinensis*, rose flowers, plum flowers, peach flowers and Chinese chives flowers 30 grams each; walnutkernels 240 grams; millet wine and spirits 2,500 grams each.

Pharmaceutical Process:

Put the flowers and kernels into a silk bag, tie up the mouth and hang it in a jar. Add the wine and the spirits, seal up the jar and let the flowers and kernels infuse for a month.

Actions:

Nourishes the kidneys, controls nocturnal emission, strengthens *yang* and cures impotence.

Indications:

Deficiency of the kidney-*yang*, impotence, dribbling urination, male sterility due to deficiency of *yang* and female sterility due to deficiency of *yin*.

Administration and Dosage:

Oral administration.

Source:

Unveiling Mysteries of Eubiotics

42. Spirit of Chinese Caterpillar Fungus

Ingredients:

Chinese caterpillar fungus 20 grams.

Pharmaceutical Process:

Grind the fungus and let it infuse in 1,000 grams of spirits for half a month.

Actions:

Nourishes the kidneys and moistens the lungs.

Indications:

Impotence, spermatorrhea, phthisical cough, expectoration of blood-tinged sputum and deuteropathic debilitation.

Administration and Dosage:

10ml in the evening.

Source:

Medicinal Nourishment and Dietetic Nourishment

43. Spirit of Seahorse

Ingredients:

Ursine seal's penis and testes, dog kidneys, donkey kidneys, seahorse 6 grams, spirits 1,000ml.

Pharmaceutical Process:

Let the organs infuse in the spirits for 7—10 days.

Indication:

Impotence.

Administration and Dosage:

15-20ml immediately after getting up in the morning.

Source:

1,100 *Folk Prescriptions of Dietetic Therapy*, 1992, p. 98.

44. Spirit of Ginseng and Pilose Antler

Ingredients:

Ginseng and pilose antler 10 grams each; fruit of Chinese wolfberry 30 grams, eucommia bark 20 grams, spirits 500ml.

Pharmaceutical Process:

Let the ginseng, antler, wolfberry fruit and eucommia bark infuse in the spirits for 7-10 days.

Indication:

Impotence.

Administration and Dosage:

15-20ml after getting up in the morning.

Source:

1,100 *Folk Prescriptions of Dietetic Therapy*, 1992, p. 98.

Section Thirty   Sterility

The sterility of a married couple living together for over 3 years without using contraceptives is called "primary sterility," and that of a married couple that remain sterile without using contraceptives 3 years after giving birth to a child or having an abortion is called "secondary sterility." Sterility can be attributed to either the husband or the wife, so both the husband and the wife should see the doctor in order to find out who is infertile.

1. Sterility Spirit

Ingredients:

Glabrous greenbrier rhizome 100 grams, stoned jujube fruit 50 grams, walnut kernels 36 grams, astragalus root; root of *Codonopsis pilosula*, rhizome of large-headed atractylodes, Chinese angelica root, rhizome of Ligusticum Chuanxiong, parched root of herbaceous peony, rhizome of rehmannia, prepared rhizome of rehmannia, aniseed, fruit of Chinese rasberry, dried orange peel, resinous wood of *Aquilaria sinensis*, aucklandia root, fruit of Chinese wolfberry, bark of *Cinnamomum cassia*, amomum fruit, frankincense, myrrh, fruit of Chinese magnoliavine and licorice root 6 grams each; honey 600 grams, spirits 2,000 grams, millet wine 1,000 grams.

Pharmaceutical Process:

Let the herbs and fruit infuse in the spirits and wine for 15 days.

Actions:

Cures sterility, regulates menstruation and protects primordial *qi*.

Indication:

Sterility.

Administration and Dosage:

Twice per day and 30ml each time.

Source:

218

2. Spirit of Chinese Angelica

Ingredients:

Chinese angelica, root of narrow-leaved polygala 75 grams each; spirits 2,500 grams.

Pharmaceutical Process:

Let the herbs infuse in the spirits for 7 days.

Indication:

Sterility.

Administration and Dosage:

15ml in the evening while it is warm.

Source:

Chunjiaoji

3. Spirit of Chinese Angelica

Ingredients:

Chinese angelica root 20 grams, safflower 10 grams.

Pharmaceutical Process:

Let the herbs infuse in 50ml of spirits of 50% alcohol content for 48 hours; filtrate the infusion and add spirits to increase the quantity of the filtrate to 100ml.

Indications:

Menoxenia, dysmenorrhea, aplasia of the womb and sterility.

Administration and Dosage:

3ml doses, 3 times after meals.

Source:

Medical Information of Shanxi.

Section Thirty-one   Gynecopathy

1. Spirit of *Erigeron Elongatus Ledeb*

Ingredient:

   Erigeron elongatus Ledab. 30 grams.

Pharmaceutical Process:

   Decoct the herb in a litre of spirits till half of the spirits is left.

Indications:

   Women's diseases of pathogenic wind type and abdominal twinges induced by stagnation of blood and *qi*.

Administration and Dosage:

   take it in two draughts.

Source:

   Synopsis of Prescriptions of the Golden Chamber.

2. Spirit of Honey

Ingredient:

   A little honey and yellow millet wine.

Pharmaceutical Process:

   Take the honey with the wine.

Indication:

   Women's itching rubella.

Source:

   Chinese Medicated Dietetics, 1985, p. 379.

3. Wine of Litchi

Ingredients:

   Fresh litchi fruit and mellow millet wine 1,000 grams each.

Pharmaceutical Process:

220

Infuse the peeled fruit in the wine for 7 days.

Indication:

Hysteroptosis.

Administration and Dosage:

15-30ml doses, twice per day.

Source:

1,1000 *Folk Prescriptions of Dietetic Therapy*, 1992, p. 232.

Section Thirty-two   Menoxenia

Menoxenia refers to abnormal menses or irregular menstrual cycle.

1. Wine of Rose Roots

Ingredients:

Rose roots 6—10 grams, yellow wine and brown sugar *q. s.*

Pharmaceutical Process:

Decoct the roots and add the wine and sugar while the decoction is still hot.

Indication:

Menoxenia.

Administration and Dosage:

Once in the morning and the evening.

Source:

Food, Chinese Medicine and Folk Prescriptions

2. Wine of Donkey-Hide Gelatin

Ingredients:

Donkey-hide gelatin 6 grams, yellow millet wine 50 ml.

Pharmaceutical Process:

Parch the gelatin with the shell powder of *Mactra quadran-*

gularis Deshayes, grind it into fine powder and mix it and the wine and warm boiled water.

Actions:

Replenishes blood and regulates menstruation.

Indications:

Scanty and pale menstruation, pain in the lower abdomen and general debilitation.

Administration and Dosage:

Take it in one draught.

Source:

Company of Chinese Medicinal Herbs of Chengdu, *Chinese Medicated Dietetics*, 1985, p. 45.

3. Wine of Black Soybeans and Eggs

Ingredients:

Black soybeans 60 grams, two eggs, millet wine 120 grams.

Pharmaceutical Process:

Decoct the soybeans and the eggs over a slow fire When the eggs are done, shell them and boil them again.

Actions:

Nourishes *qi* and blood, dispels cold and regulates menstruation.

Indications:

Deficiency, cold and dysmenorrhea and delayed menstrual period.

Administration and Dosage:

Eat the eggs and drink the decoction with the wine.

Source:

Company of Chinese Medicinal Herbs of Chengdu, *Chinese*

Medicated Dietetics, 1985, p. 45.

Section-thirty Three   Dysmenorrhea

Dysmenorrhea refers to abdominal pain and lumbago, sometimes sharp and even unbearable, with concomitant pallor, cold sweat, cold hands and feet, nausea and vomiting before, during or after menstruation.

1. Wine of Walnuts

Ingredients:

Walnuts 500 grams, yellow millet wine 1,000ml, brown sugar 250 grams.

Pharmaceutical Process:

Pound the walnut shells into small pieces, put them into a container, add the wine and seal it up. Filtrate the infusion after 20-30 days, add the sugar and melt it in the filtrate. Then pour the filtrate into a bottle.

Indication:

Dysmenorrhea due to deficiency of the liver and kidneys.

Administration and Dosage:

10ml doses, twice per day. 7 days constitute a course of treatment. Begin taking it 5 days before menstruation.

Source:

Chinese Medicated Dietetics, p. 311

2. Spirit of Chinese Angelica and Astragalus

Ingredients:

Chinese angelica root and astragalus root 150 grams each, jujube fruit 100 grams, spirits 500ml.

Pharmaceutical Process:

Wash the roots and fruit clean, put them into a silk bag and let them infuse in the spirits in a sealed container.

Indication:

Dysmenorrhea due to deficiency of *qi* and blood.

Administration and Dosage:

10ml doses, twice per day. 7 days constitute a course of treatment. Begin taking it 5 days before menstruation.

Source:

Chinese Medicated Dietetics, p. 311.

3. Spirit of Motherwort

Ingredient:

Motherwort 30 grams.

Pharmaceutical Process:

Add water and spirits of equal quantity to the herb and decoct it.

Indication:

Pain induced by blood stagnation.

Administration and Dosage:

Take it in one draught.

Source:

Chinese Medicated Dietetics, 1985, p. 264.

Section Thirty-Four   Amenia

If a woman of eighteen or over fails to have a menstrual onset or has a cessation of the menses for over 3 months, she is said to be suffering from amenia, which is divided into primary and secondary stages.

1. Spirit of Achyranthes, Ginseng and Chinese Angelica

Ingredients:

Achyranthes root 30 grams, nutgrass flatsedge rhizome, pilose asiabell root and Chinese angelica root 15 grams each; safflower 9 grams, cassia bark 9 grams.

Pharmaceutical Process:

Mince the herbs and let them infuse in 500 grams of spirits for 7 days.

Actions:

Promotes the flow of *qi* and blood, nourishes blood and regulates menstruation.

Indication:

Anemia.

Administration and Dosage:

5-10ml in the morning and 10-20ml in the evening till the onset of the menses. Those with strong constitutions can increase the dosage to 20-30ml and shorten the duration of treatment.

Cautions:

Pregnant women and women with heart trouble, bronchial asthma and leukorrhea must not take it.

Source:

News Reports on Chinese Medicinal Herbs of Sichuan, Issue 1, 1977, p. 46.

2. Wine of Mulberry Fruit

Ingredients:

Mulberry fruit 15 grams, safflower 3 grams, spatholobus stem 12 grams, yellow millet wine.

Pharmaceutical Process:

Decoct the herbs in water and a little wine.

Indication:

Amenia.

Administration and Dosage:

twice per day.

Source:

A Handbook of Family Dietetic Therapy, 1982, p. 152.

3. Spirit of Spatholobus

Ingredients:

Spatholobus stem and rock candy 60 grams each; spirits 500 grams.

Pharmaceutical Process:

Let the herb and candy infuse in the spirits for 7 days.

Actions:

Promotes blood circulation, replenishes blood and removes obstruction in the collaterals and channels.

Indications:

Blood stagnation, anemia and traumatic injury.

Administration and Dosage:

Twice per day and 10ml each time.

Source:

Chinese Medicated Dietetics, 1985, p. 203.

Section Thirty-five   Leukorrhea

The sticky liquid like mucous or saliva flowing from the vagina is usually called "whites. " If it flows in large quantities, or its color, quality and smell have pathogenic changes or accompany certain general symptoms, the disease is called leukorrhea.

1. Spirit of Turtle Glue

Ingredient:

glue of soft-shelled turtle 9 grams.

Pharmaceutical Process:

Dissolve it in spirits and take it in the morning.

Indication:

Incessant whites.

Source:

Chinese Medicated Dietetics, 1985, p. 215

Section Thirty-six   Edema of Pregnancy

Edema of pregnancy is swelling of the face or limbs during pregnancy.

1. Wine of Tangerine Peel

Ingredient:

Tangerine peel 120 grams.

Pharmaceutical Process:

Wash the peel clean, grind it into powder and mix six gram portions with a certain amount of yellow millet wine.

Indication:

Edema of pregnancy induced by *qi* stagnation.

Administration and Dosage:

3 times per day. 7 days constitute a course of treatment.

Source:

Chinese Dietetic Therapeutics, p. 316.

Section Thirty-seven   Postpartum Diseases

Postpartum diseases mainly include pain in the lower abdomen.

1. Spirit of Black-Boned Chicken

Ingredients:

Dried *Gallus gallus domesticus*, Chinese angelica root, rhizome of Ligusticum Chunaxiong, noterpterygium root, root of *Pterospermum heterophyllum Hance*, root of Dahurian angelica, maganolia bark, safflower, dried ginger, root of *Codonopsis pilosula*, astragalus root, Chinese yam, jujube fruit, root of herbaceous peony, fruit of Chinese wolfberry, chichen claws, pork tendons.

Actions:

Dispels cold, promotes blood circulation, replenishes *qi* and nourishes blood.

Indications:

Numbness of the hands and feet and soreness and pains in the waist and knees due to pathogenic wind; cold and dampness and postpartum deficiency of *qi* and blood, the clinical symptoms of which are soreness and pains in the waist and knees which worsen when it is cold, numbness of the hands and feet, pale or sallow face, pale and enlarged tongue with white, greasy or slimy fur and deep, thready and slow pulse.

Administration and Dosage:

Oral administration, 30-50ml doses, once or twice per day.

Caution:

Those with a fever or a sore throat must not not take it.

Source:

Pharmaceutical Factory No. 1 of Foshan City, Guangdong, Medicinal standards of Guangdong Province in *Basic Preparations of Chinese Medicine*, Vol. 1, 1988, p. 317.

2. Spirit of Black-Boned Chicken

Ingredients:

Dried *Gallus gallus domesticus* 160 grams (or fresh *Gallus gallus domesticus* 320 grams, cleaned); Chinese angelica root, root of Ligusticum Chuanxiong, safflower, rhizome of homalomana 160 grams each, root of herbaceous peony and peach kernels 15 grams, *Poria cocos* 20 grams.

Pharmaceutical Process:

Steam the dried chicken for 15 minutes, let it cool down, then let it infuse in spirit for 25 days. Put it together with the other ingredients into a container, add spirits, seal up the container, let them infuse for 45-55 days and then filtrate them. The spirit needed altogether amounts to 16,960ml.

Actions:

Warms the channels and collaterals, dispels wind, promotes blood circulation and dissipates blood stasis.

Indication:

Postpartum dizziness, pains and weakness of the limbs and dysmenorrhea.

Administration and Dosage:

Oral administration, 15-30ml doses, 3-4 times per day.

Cautions:

Those with a cold, or a fever, or a sore throat or conjunctival congestion should not take it.

Source:

Pharmacopoiea of the People's Republic of China, Vol. 1, 1977, p. 717.

3. Wine of Brown Sugar

Ingredients:

Brown sugar *q. s.* , yellow millet wine 250 grams.

Pharmaceutical Process:

Bring the wine to the boil, add the sugar and boil it for another 2-3 minutes.

Indication:

Postpartum simple loose stool.

Administration and Dosage:

Take it at a draught.

Source:

Chinese Medicated Dietetics, 1985, p. 379.

4. Spirit of *Celosia Cristata*

Ingredients:

Dried spike of Celosia cristata 15 grams, spirits *q. s.*

Pharmaceutical Process:

Decoct them.

Indications:

Postpartum pain due to blood stagnation or diarrhea.

Administration and Dosage:

Take it at a draught.

Source:

Chinese Medicated Dietetics, 1985, p. 261.

5. Wine of Rehmannia and Motherwort

Ingredients:

Rhizome of rehmannia 6 grams, motherwort 10 grams, yellow millet wine 200 ml.

Pharmaceutical Process:

Steam them in a cup for 20 minutes.

Indications:

Postpartum blood stasis and abdominal pain.

Administration and Dosage:

50ml doses, twice per day. Take it while it is warm.

Source:

Chinese Medicated Dietetics, 1985, p. 272.

6. Wine of Rice Fermented with Red Yeast

Ingredients:

Rice fermented with red yeast 10-12 grams, yellow millet wine *q. s.*

Pharmaceutical Process:

Decoct them.

Indications:

Postpartum blood stagnation and abdominal pain.

Administration and Dosage:

Take it while it is warm.

Source:

Food, Chinese Medicine and Folk Prescriptions.

7. Spirit of Black Soybeans

Ingredients:

Black soybeans 500 grams, spirits 1,000 grams.

Pharmaceutical Process:

Parch the beans till they turn purple, put them into the spirit, remove the beans when the spirits turn dark purple.

Actions:

Dissipates blood stasis, dispels wind and heat.

Administration and Dosage:

Oral administration according to individual capacity for spirits.

Source:

Chinese Medicated Spirit, 1985, p. 280.

8. Spirit of Honey

Ingredients:

Honey 60 grams, juice of rhizome of rehmannia 50 grams, millet wine 100ml.

Pharmaceutical Process:

Bring the juice and spirits to the boil 5 times in a copper container and mix them and the honey.

Actions:

Promotes blood circulation and dissipates blood stasis.

Indications:

Metrorrhagia after an abortion and dysmenorrhea due to blood stasis.

Administration and Dosage:

Divide the spirits into two doses.

Source:

Proven Prescriptions.

Section Thirty-eight   Acute Mastitis

Acute mastitis occurs in the breasts. Its clinical symptoms are hard lumps, swelling pain and a sensation of burning heat in the breasts, a fever and aversion to cold. The lumps take shape within a week and suppurate 10 days later.

1. Spirit of *Sonechus Oleraceus L.*

Ingredients:

Fresh *Sonechus oleracleus L.* 90 grams, spirits 120 grams.

Pharmaceutical Process:

Wash the herb clean, put it and the spirits into a pot, add about 800-1,000ml of water and decoct them for about half an hour.

Indication:

Mastitis in initial stage.

Administration and Dosage:

150-200ml doses, twice per day.

Source:

1,100 *Folk Prescriptions of Dietetic Therapy*, 1992, p. 182.

Section Thirty-nine   Dermatosis

1. Spirit of Dittany Bark

Ingredient:

Dittany bark 150 grams.

Pharmaceutical Process:

Let the bark infuse in 500 grams of spirits for 3 days.

Actions:

Dispels heat, wind and dampness and toxic material.

Indications:

Senile chronic bronchitis, eczema and scabies, etc.

Administration and Dosage:

Oral administration, 10ml doses, 3 times per day.

Source: *Weifang Medicine*, Issue 1,1972, p. 26.

2. Antipruritic Spirit

Ingredients:

Dittany bark, fruiting aerial parts of wormseed goosefoot and flavescent sophora root 150 grams each; spirit *q. s.*

Pharmaceutical Process:

Pound the herbs and let them infuse in the spirits in a covered container for 7-14 days. Filtrate the infusion, press the dregs to obtain extract and mix it with the filtrate. Keep the mixture static for 24 hours, then filtrate it and add spirit to increase the quantity of the filtrate to 1,000ml.

Actions:

Antiseptic and antipruritic.

Administration and Dosage:

Apply it topically.

Storage:

Keep it airtight.

Source:

College of Pharmacy of Shenyang, *Common Pharmaceutical Preparations*, 1975, p. 164.

3. Composite Spirit of Cnidum Fruit

Ingredients:

Cnidum fruit and flavescent sophora root 248 grams each; fruiting aerial parts of wormseed goosefoot 150 grams; alum, ledebouriella root and dittany bark 124 grams each; spirits 4,000 ml.

Pharmaceutical Process:

Pound the herbs and alum, add 400ml of the spirits and let them infuse in the spirits in a sealed container for 30 days. Stir them once a day in the first 7 days and once a week in the remaining days. Obtain clear liquid from the infusion, press the dregs, filtrate them, then mix the clear liquid and the filtrate. Keep the mixture static for some time and filtrate it. The filtrate is a brown-red liquid.

Actions:

Dispels dampness and relieves itching.

Indications:

Neurodermatitis, cutaneous pruritis, chronic eczema, flat wart, and pompholyx.

Administration and Dosage:

Apply it topically 2-3 times per day.

Storage:

Keep it airtight in a dark, cool and dry place.

Source:

A Handbook of Shanxi Pharmaceutical Preparations, 1976, p. 119.

4. Psoriasis Spirit No. 1

Ingredients:

Bletilla tuber, goldenlarch bark, areca seed, stemona root and Sichuan peppers 500 grams each; chaulmoogra seed 250 grams, Chinese blistering beetles (without wings and legs) 100 grams, salicylic acid, benzonic acid.

Pharmaceutical Process:

Pound and crush the first five ingredients respectively and put them into a percolator with the powder at the bottom and the small pieces on top. Grind the beetles into powder, mix it and the seed of chaulmoogra, then pound the mixture into paste. Put it on top of the pounded herbs mentioned above, cover them with a board with holes in it and submerge them in spirits of 60—73% alcohol content or alcohol. The spirit should be a few centimeters above the herbs. Cover the percolator, let the herbs infuse in the spirits for 5-7 days, then percolate them using 15,000ml of spirits in all. Add 5% of solicylic acid and 10% of benzonic acid to the percolate and mix them.

Actions:

Softens hard lumps and subdues them, destroys parasites and relieves the itch.

Indications:

Neurodermatitis, tinea manuum and timea pedis.

Administration:

Apply it to the affected part.

Caution:

Do not use it when the disease is in the acute stage.

Source:

Hospital No. 1 and Hospital No. 2 attached to Xian Medical College, *A Handbook of Pharmaceutical Preparations for Dermatosis*, 1977

5. Spirit of Goldenlarch Bark

Ingredients:

Goldenlarch bark, arisaema tuber and areca seed 30 grams each; seed of *Momordica cochinchinensis Spr.* and camphor 15 grams each; thirty Chinese blistering beetles, toad venom 9 grams.

Pharmaceutical Process:

Grind them into small pieces and let them infuse in 500 grams of spirits.

Indication:

Tinea.

Administration and Dosage:

Apply it to the affected part.

Source:

Encyclopedia of Diagnosis and Treatment of External Diseases.

6. Spirit of Chinese Gall and Alum

Ingredients:

Chinese gall 250 grams, alum 100-200 grams.

Pharmaceutical Process:

Let them infuse in 1,000 grams of spirit for 5—7 days, filtrate the infusion and remove the dregs.

Actions:

Astringent, antipruritic and preventive.

Indication:

Rice field dermatosis.

Administration and Dosage:

Apply it to the hands, feet and shanks before labouring in rice fields.

Source:

Hospital No. 1 and Hospital No. 2 attached to Xian Medical College, *A Handbook of Pharmaceutical Preparations for Dermatosis*, 1977

7. Spirit of Snakes

Ingredients:

Long-noded pit vipers and *Bungarus fasciatus* 2,500 grams each; *Zaocysd humnaeds* 10,000 grams, cobras and tetrandra roots 5,000 grams each; inflorescence of *Rhododendron molle G. Don* 125,000 grams, *Schefflera arboricola Hayata* 5,000 grams, *Photinia serrulata* 25,000 grams, spatholobus stems 5,000 grams, common St. Paulswort 5,000 grams, *Schizophragma int-*

grifolium 5,000 grams.

Pharmaceutical Process:

Wash the ingredients clean, drip-dry them, cut them into small pieces and let them infuse in 250,000 grams of 73% proof spirits in a sealed container for a year.

Actions:

Dispels wind, relieves itching, removes obstruction in the channels and collaterals and nourishes the skin.

Indication:

Psoriasis.

Administration and Dosage:

Oral administration, 9—15 gram doses before or after meals, 2—3 times per day. Those who cannot drink can dilute the spirits with cold boiled water before taking it. For external use, 2—3 times per day. Dip a little absorbent cotten in the medicated spirit, apply it topically to the affected part, cover it with plastic film or paper and then fix it with adhesive.

Source:

Journal of Hunan Medicine, No. 6, 1977, p. 29

8. Corn Plaster

Ingredients:

Salicylic acid 85 grams, benzonic acid 10 grams, sulfanamide 2-3 grams, procaine 1-3 grams, camphor ball 0.2 gram, white sugar q. s., spirits *q. s.*

Pharmaceutical Process:

Grind all the ingredients except the spirits, sift them, mix them, put them into a clean bottle, add the spirits and seal up the bottle.

Actions:

Erodes diseased flesh and cutin and relieves inflammation to stop pain.

Indicatinos:

Corn and callus.

Administration and Dosage:

Soak the affected part in warm water and dry it . Cut a hole slightly bigger than the corn in a piece of adhesive tape and stick the tape around the corn to protect the surrounding skin. Apply a little of the plaster on the corn . If the corn is on the sole, make a thin cord by rolling absorbent cotten between the palms and wrap it round the plaster to prevent it from spilling; stick a piece of adhesive tape on it to fix it. Take off the tape a week later and scrape the light grey part with a sharpened tool (e. g. a bone or bamboo stick), taking out the root if the corn is small, or repeating the treatment if the corn is big and cannot be cured easily.

Source:

Changwei, Shandong Province, *The Barefoot Doctor*, Issue 5, 1977 , p. 16.

9. Spirit of *Cuscuta Chinensis*

Ingredients:

Fresh *Cuscuta chinensis* 300 grams.

Pharmaceutical Process:

Let the whole herbs infuse in 600 grams of spirits of 75% alcohol content for 5-7 days, then filtrate the infusion and remove the dregs.

Action:

Dispels wind.

Indication:

Leukoderma.

Administration:

Apply it to the diseased part.

Cautions:

Those ill with acute inflammation or allergic to it must not use it.

Source:

Hospital No. 1 and Hospital No. 2 attached to Xian Medical College, *A Handbook of Pharmaceutical Preparations for Dermatosis*, 1977

10. Spirit of Chinese Ephedra

Ingredients:

Chinese ephedra and roots of Chinese ephedra 60 grams each, 5 cans of spirits.

Pharmaceutical Process:

Decoct the herbs in the spirits for a duration in which 3 joss sticks can be burnt up in succession and leave the decoction uncovered for a night.

Indication:

Brandy nose.

Administration and Dosage:

Oral administration , 30-50ml doses in the morning and evening.

Source:

The Golden Mirror of Medicine

11. Spirit of Pallas-Pit Viper and *Viola Yedoensis Mak*

Ingredients:

One or two pallas-pit vipers, 30 grams of *Viola yedoensis Mak.*

Pharmaceutical Process:

Put the live snakes, 1, 000ml of spirits of 60% alcohol content and *Viola yedonesis Mak.* into a bottle. Seal it up, put it in a dark and cool place and use it at least 3 months later. The longer the duration of infusion, the better. Replenish the bottle with no more than 1, 000ml of spirits when the original medicinal spirits are used up.

Actions:

Dispels heat and relieves inflammation.

Indication:

Suppurative infection of the soft tissues.

Administration and Dosage:

Dip absorbent cotten in the spirits, apply it to the affected part and put plastic film over the cotten. If the injury is on a finger or a toe, the finger from a used rubber glove can be used. Change the dressing several times a day to ensure that the cotten on the affected part is wet with medicinal spirits.

Source:

New Medicine, Issue 5, 1974, p. 249.

12. Spirit of Chinese Blistering Beetles

Ingredients:

20-30 Chinese blistering beetles, goldenlarch bark and camphor powder 9 grams each; spiris of 45—60 alcohol content 150 grams.

Pharmaceutical Process:

Let the minced beetles and bark infuse in the spirits separately for 1-2 weeks. Remove the dregs, mix the infusions, add the camphor powder and filtrate the mixture.

Indication:

Neurodermatitis.

Administration and Dosage:

Wash the affected part clean, apply a little of the spirits to it and repeat the step 10 minutes later. Do twice per day. Use the spirits for 1-3 weeks.

Lotion:

Tea (stored for over a year) and old Chinese mugwort leaves 15 grams each; old ginger (mashed) 30 grams, two bulbs of purple-skinned garlic (mashed), a little edible salt.

Pharmaceutical Process:

Decoct the ingredients.

Administration and Dosage:

One dose every two days after the medicated spirit is applied to the affeted part. Wash the affected part twice per day for 1-3 weeks when a scab forms over it.

Source:

Chenzhou Prefectural People's Hospital, Hunan Province, *Selection of the Materials of the National Exhibition of Chinese Medicinal Herbs and New Therapy*, 1972, p. 364.

13. Wine of Honey

Ingredients:

Honey made from narrow-leaved oleaster flowers 500 grams, cooked glutinous rice 2 kilograms, distiller's yeast 250 grams, boiled water 5 *kilograms*.

Pharmaceutical Process:

Put the ingredients into a bottle and keep them airtight for 7 days.

Indication:

Rubella.

Administration and Dosage:

Oral administration.

Source:

A Handbook of Family Dietetic Therapy, 1982, p, 514.

14. Spirit of Pallas-Pit Viper

Ingredient:

Pallas-pit viper.

Pharmaceutical Process:

Put the live snake and two decalitres of good spirits into a container, seal it up, bury it in a place often soaked with horse urine and dig it out a year later.

Indications:

Malignant sores, epilepsy and stubborn arthralgia.

Administration and Dosage:

30-50 ml. each time.

Source:

A Handbook of Family Dietetic Therapy, 1982, p. 516.

15. Wine of Sweet Wormseed

Ingredients:

Sweet wormseed leaves 200 grams, glutinous rice.

Pharmaceutical Process:

Boil the rice, mix it with the juice of the leaves and distiller's yeast to make wine.

Actions:

Dispels heat and cools blood.

Indication:

Lupus erythematosus.

Administration and Dosage:

50ml doese, twice per day.

Source:

Proven Prescriptions

Section Forty   Bleeding

1. Wine of Pine Pollen

Ingredients:

Pine pollen 500 grams, rice wine 1,500 grams.

Pharmaceutical Process:

Put the pollen into a bag and let it infuse in the wine for 5 days.

Actions:

Astringent and restringent.

Indication:

Traumatic bleeding.

Administration and Dosage:

20ml. doses, twice per day.

Source:

Yuanhejiyongjing.

Section Forty-one   *Alopecia Areata*

Alopecia areata refers to sudden local baldness and has no conscious symptoms.

1. Spirit of Cayenne

Ingredients:

Cayenne 10 grams, spirits 50 grams.

Pharmaceutical Process:

Cut the cayenne into thin strips, let them infuse in the spirits for 10 days, then filtrate the infusion to remove the dregs.

Indication:

Alopecia areata.

Administration and Dosage:

Apply it to the bald part several times per day.

Source:

A Handbook of Family Dietetic Therapy, 1982, p. 50.

2. Alcohol of *Biota Orientalis*

Ingredients:

Fresh leaty twig of *Biota orientalis* 30-60 grams, alcohol with a concentration of 60% *q. s.*

Pharmaceutical Process:

Let the twig infuse in the alcohol for 7 days.

Actions:

Dispels heat, cools blood and helps hair grow.

Administration and Dosage:

Apply the alcohol to the bald part 3 times per day.

Source:

Chinese Medicated Dietetics, 1985, p. 259.

Section Forty-two Beriberi

Beriberi is a recurrent disease. The patient usually has small and itching blisters between the toes and if the blisters are punctured, liquid will flow from them and then scabs will form over them.

1. Spirit of Poplar Bark

Ingredient:

Poplar bark.

Pharmaceutical Process:

Wash the bark clean, cut it into slices and decoct them in spirits.

Indications:

Pathogenic wind, beriberi and accumulation of phlegm in the hypochondrium.

Administration and Dosage:

Oral administration.

Source:

A Handbook of Family Dietetic Therapy, 1982, p. 510.

2. Wine of Atractylodes

Ingredient:

Rhizomes of Chinese atractylodes 15, 000 grams.

Pharmaceutical Process:

Wash the rhizomes clean, pound them, let them infuse in 150 kilograms of water for 20 days, remove the rhizomes and make wine from the juice and rice in a normal way.

Indications:

Sores due to wind and dampness and beriberi.

Administration and Dosage:

Oral administration.

Source:

A Handbook of Family Dietetic Therapy, 1982, p. 509.

Section Forty-three Hernia

Hernia refers to the bulging of an internal part of the body with concomitant pain due to general disorder of *qi*. It includes some diseases of the genitals, testes and scrotum.

1. Spirit of Tangerine Seed

Ingredients:

Tangerine seed 15 grams, a little spirit.

Pharmaceutical Process:

Parch and grind the seed and decoct it in the spirits.

Actions:

Regulates the flow of *qi* to stop pain.

Indications:

Hernia of the small intestine and pain of the testes.

Administrationd and Dosage:

Take it at a draught.

Source:

A Handbook of Family Dietetic Therapy, 1982, p. 138.

2. Wine of *Poncirus Trifoliata Raf.*

Ingredients:

Six fruits of *Pocirus trifoliata Raf.*, yellow millet wine 250 grams.

Pharmaceutical Process:

Let the fruits infuse in the wine.

Indications:

Hernia and swelling of the testes.

Administration and Dosage:

Oral administration, 15ml each time.

Source:

Nanjing Folk Prescriptions of Medicinal Herbs.

Section Forty-four Angititis

Angititis refers to thromboangititis obliterans, which usually attacks the lower limbs of men and can even induce gangrene.

1. Vascular Ventilation Spirit

Ingredients:

Ardisia gigantifolia root 50 grams, safflower 25 grams, *paris polyphylla* 25 grams, Chinese angelica root-tip 50 grams, loranthus mulbery misletoe 50 grams, frankincense 15 grams, clematis root 50 grams, myrrh, achyranthes root 25 grams, astragalus root 25 grams, pilose asiabell root 25 grams, honeylocust spine 25 grams, cinnamon twig 25 grams.

Pharmaceutical Process:

Let the herbs infuse in 2500—3000 grams of Sanhua spirit for three weeks.

Actions:

Dispels wind-cold, promotes blood circulation and the flow of *qi*.

Indications:

Cold and dampness, stagnancy of *qi* and blood stasis.

Caution:

In cases of damp-heat, remove dampness and pathogenic heat first to promote blood circulation and remove stasis, and take the spirits when the inflammation is under control. For heart patients, let the herbs infuse in water instead of spirits, reduce the amount of each herb by 1/10, and take one dose each time.

However, the water dose is less effective than the medicinal spirits.

Administration and Dosage:

Oral administration, 20-100ml. each time and four times per day (those with a great capacity for alcohol can exceed the dose, but do not get drunk). One month is a course of treatment and there is an interval of 3-5 days between courses.

Source:

Guangxi Hygiene Issue 6, 1974, p. 25.

2. *Bungarus Pavus* Spirit

Ingredients:

One *bungarus parvus*, one toad (with red eyes and patterns on its wrist), *lonicera confusa* 90 grams, achyranthis root 60 grams, aconite root 30 grams, spirits of 75% alcohol content 150 grams

Pharmaceutical Process:

Put the herbs and spirits together into a jar, seal it and put it into a larger container with water. Decoct the herbs for 1—1.5 hours and filtrate them when they cool down.

Indication:

Thromboangitis obliterans

Administration and Dosage:

For the first two days, one dose every day (till one gets completely drunk); from the third day on, 50—100ml doses, twice per day (depending on the patient's condition and capacity for alcohol) until recovery.

Source:

Hospital of Tangshan Steel Plant of Hebei Province

3. Vasculitis Spirits

Ingredients:

Boston ivy 350 grams, spirits 100ml

Pharmaceutical Process:

Grind the Boston ivy into fine powder, wet it with some of the spirits, put it into a container and let it infuse in the remaining spirits for seven days according to the method of extraction by cold infusion.

Actions:

Removes obstruction in collaterals and eliminates inflammation.

Contraindication:

Hypertension

Source:

Folk Preparations of Chinese Herbal Medicine of Guizhou (1977, p. 203).

Section Forty-five　Snakebite

Local swelling and continuous burning pain or numbness occur after a snakebite. Either blood or serum exudate oozes from the wound. The lymph glands nearby swell noticeably and are tender. Meanwhile there are symptoms induced by general poisoning such as pyrexia, headache, pain in the limbs, choking sensation in the chest, nausea and vomiting, dark red urine or even death in serious cases. Add other snakebite medicines to the following if necessary.

1. Snakebite Spirit I

Ingredients:

Goldthread root 6000 grams, zanthoxylum root 45,000 grams, evodiae fruit 22,000 grams *zaocys dhumnades* 17,000 grams, *evolvulus alsinoides* 17,000 grams, asarum 9000 grams, rhubarb 28,000 grams, tinospora root 17,000 grams, schizonepetae 56,000 grams, dahurian angelica root 28,000 grams, yellow-corktree bark 12,000 grams, *faeces trogopterorum* 22,000 grams, corton leaves 5000 grams, realgar 22,000 grams, dried leaves and young foliferous branches of *murraya paniculata* 34,000 grams, Haidiyingzhen 60,000 grams, *rehmannia glutinosa* 40,000 grams, *molsa cavaleriei* 40,000 grams, node of lotus rhizome 56,000 grams

Pharmaceutical Process:

Pound and mix 2/3 of the above herbs and let them infuse in 1000 kilograms of spirits for 20 days. Filtrate the infusion, and let the remaining herbs infuse in the filtrate for 25 days. Filtrate the second infusion.

Actions:

Removes toxic materials and relieves swelling

Indication:

Snakebite

Administration and Dosage:

Oral administration, 30ml. once per day for slight cases, 60ml every two or three hours for severe cases. For external use, dip cotton cloth or paper in the spirit and apply it on the affected part after cutting open the wound and rubbing it gently with garlic head or chili from up to down till it bleeds.

Source:

Selection of Materials of National Exhibition of Chinese

Herbal Medicine and New Therapy (People's Hospital of Xinhui county , Guangdong Province)

2. Snakebite Spirit II

Ingredients:

Hyacinth bean, notoginseng, root of *christia vespertilionis*, *sapindus mukorrossi* bark, Chinese sapium bark, *iris speculatrix* 15 grams each.

Pharmaceutical Process:

Clean, dry and mince the above herbs, let them infuse in 500 grams of rice wine for one month and filtrate them to remove the dregs.

Actions:

Removes pathogenic heat and toxic materials, induces diuresis and removes swelling

Indication:

Snakebite

Administration and Dosage:

Oral administration, 30-50ml doses for adults; double doses for severe cases. People bitten by *Bungarus fasciatus* or *Bungarus multicinctus* take one does every half an hour and then one dose every two or three hours after getting better with three doses. People bitten by *Trimeresurus stejnegeri* or Naja naja take one dose every two or three hours--one dose every half hour for severe cases and one dose every two or three hours after getting better. Also, one can apply the spirit to the affected part from up to down four times per day; women and children can take it with warm water.

Source:

New Medicine (People's Hospital of Huang County, Guangxi Province)

3. Snake Spirit I

Ingredients:

Chlorophytum laxuam 200 grams

Pharmaceutical Process:

Let the herb infuse in 500 grams of rice wine of 40% alcohol content for two weeks

Action:

Removes pathogenic heat from the blood

Indications:

Snakebite, swelling pain caused by traumatic injuries, pus and abcess

Administration and Dosage:

Oral administration, 20-40ml. doses.

Source:

Selection of Materials of National Exhibition of Chinese Herbal Medicine and New Therapy (People's Hospital of Zhong shan County, Guangdong Province)

Remarks:

The spirit is effective for snakebite by *Bungarus multicinctus*, but when the snakebite causes central nervous system symptoms, proper comprehensive treatment is needed.

4. Snake Spirit II

Ingredients:

Isodon amethystoides 60 grams, *cynanchum paniculatum* root and rice wine (or Sanhua rice wine) 15 grams each.

Pharmaceutical Process:

Let the herbs infuse together in the rice wine for three weeks

Actions:

Removes pathogenic heat, toxic materials, swelling and blood stagnancy

Indication:

Snakebite

Administration and Dosage:

Oral administration. 50-100ml doses first then 25-50ml doses three or four times per day for three or four days

Side-Effect:

Emesis occurs to some particular patients

Source:

Medical Scientific and technological Information (Issue 2, 1972, P. 1. Guangxi)

5. Composite Hyacinth Bean Spirit

Ingredients:

Hyacinth bean, *polygala telephioides*, *tylophora floribunda*, *sapindus mukorossi* rootand Chinese sapium root 15 grams, *iris speculatrix* 9 grams

Pharmaceutical Process:

Cut the above herbs to pieces and let them infuse in 500 grams of spirits for 20 days

Actions:

Removes pathogenic heat, toxic materials, swelling and pain

Indication:

Snakebite

Administration and Dosage:

Oral administration, two spoons every hour, three or four times per day for adults; children should take smaller doses

Source:

Collection of Chinese Herbal Medicine Vol. 1, 1973, P. 111

6. Realgar Snakebite Spirit

Ingredients:

Realgar, chuanxiong rhizome and ledebouriella root 18 grams each; liquorice root 6 grams; safflower and asarum 15 gramseach; *faeces trogop-terorum* 3 grams; Sichuan aconite root, *ophioglossum vulgatum* 6 grams and wild aconite root 6 grams each; *juncus setchuensis*, *alocasis cucullata* root, *sagittaria trifolia*, *polygonum perfoliatum* 9 grams each.

Pharmaceutical Process:

Let the above herbs infuse in spirit for 7 days

Indication:

Snakebite

Administration and Dosage:

Oral administration, 10-20ml doses; or apply the spirits to the wound or to the bare parts for prevention

Source:

Selection of Materials of National Exhibition of Chinese Herbal Medicine and New Therapy (1972, P. 257, Yanjin Medicine Company of Zhaotong prefecture, Yunnan Province)

7. Short Tube Lycoris Spirit

Ingredients:

Short-tube lycoris, *tinospora sagittata*, *zaocys dhumnades*, *hemiboea subcapitata*, dried stem of *sargentodoxae cuneata*, *ophioglossum vulgatum*, *metaolexis japonia*, Huyacao, *herminium monorehis*, Lanshefeng, *aconitum sinomontanum* root, *spiranthes sinensis*, clematis root, *clematis armandi* and Mojiazicao 9 grams each; *ardisia frevicaulis* root, licorice root and dahurian angelica root 6 grams each; safflower and asarum 3 grams each.

Pharmaceutical Process:

Let all the above herbs infuse in 1500 grams of fine quality spirits for 7 days and remove the dregs from the infusion

Administration and Dosage:

Oral administration 100-200 gram doses; or apply the dregs to the wound for external treatment

Source:

Selection of Materials of National Exhibition of Chinese Herbal Medicine and New Therapy (1972. P. 256, Zhuxi County, Hunan Province)

Remarks:

It is locally considered that each dose can prevent snakebite for two years.

8. *Oldenlandiae Diffusae* Spirit

Ingredients:

Oldenlandiae diffusae 2 leaves; *hypericum japonicum*, *rostellularia procumbens*, *eclipta*, red Tianwu, white Tianwu and *lindania anagallis* 30 grams each

Pharmaceutical Process:

Wash, clean and pound the herbs, wring 70% of the juice out of them and mix the juice with rice wine of equal amount

Indication:

Snakebite

Administration and Dosage:

Oral administration once per day, two or three doses for slight cases and three to five doses for severe cases; or apply the dregs to the wound and the swelling for external treatment.
Source:

Selection of Materials of National Exhibition of Chinese Herbal Medicine and New Therapy (1972, P. 262. People's Hospital of Tongan County, Fujian Province).

9. *Diyouzi* Spirit

Ingredients:

Fresh *Diyouzi* 5-6grams, *cynanchum paniculata* 2-3grams.

Pharmaceutical Process:

Pound the above herbs and let them infuse in spirits for several minutes

Indication:

Snakebite

Administration and Dosage:

5-10ml for oral administration; or cut hair from the *anterior front* and rub the skin to make it bleed, apply the dregs to it and change the dressing every day; apply the dregs to the wound if there is pain.

Source:

Selection of Materials of National Exhibition of Chinese Herbal Medicine and New Therapy (1972. P. 260, People's Hospital of Fujian Province).

10. Snakebite Wine I

Ingredients:

Zanthoxulum root and *euodialepta* 45 grams each; hypernicum and *pteris semipinnata* 24 grams, *lobeliae chinensis*.

Pharmaceutical Process:

Let the above herbs infuse in rice wine of 40% alcohol content for one month (or for ten days in an emergency)

Actions:

Removes pathogenic heat and toxic materials

Indication:

Snakebite

Administration and Dosage:

Oral administration: 24-30 grams for adults, 15 grams for children. External use: dip absorbent cotton in the wine and apply it to the wounded part.

Source:

News Reports on New Medicine (Issue 3, 1977, P. 61).

11. Snakebite Spirit Ⅱ

Ingredients:

Wikstromia root 90 grams, shiny prickly ash root 120 grams, Xialayangen 60—90 grams, ecdysanthera root 60 grams

Pharmaceutical Process:

Let all the herbs infuse in rice wine of 30% alcohol content for 7—10 days

Actions:

Removes pathogenic heat and toxic materials

Indication:

Snakebite

Administration and Dosage:

Oral administration: 10ml doses, 2 or 3 times per day. External use: disinfect the affected part, cut open the wound and drain off the toxic substances, then apply the wine from around the edge to the wound's center four or five times per day

Source:

News Reports on New Medicine (Issue 31, 1977, P. 61)

Section Forty-six Fracture

A fracture is usually caused by external injury which leads to broken bones. It is divided into closed and open fractures.

1. Bone-Reunion Spirit

External Treatment

Ingredients:

Green *vitis vinifera* root 5 kilograms, *torricellia angulata* leaves 1.5 kilograms, *ampelopsis humulifolia* leaves 1.5 kilograms, *elshoizia penduliflora* 1.5 kilograms, root and leaves of *euonymus fortunei* 2.5 kilograms, *tetrastigma hypoglaucum* 2.5 kilograms, *toddalia asiatica* root 1 kilogram, *solanum verbasaifolium* leaves 3 kilograms, *helwingia japonica* root 2 kilograms, *potentilla freyniana* leaves 2 kilograms

Pharmaceutical Process:

Grind the herbs into fine powder, wet part of the powder with spirits, then mix it with water into paste

Indication:

Fracture

Administration and Dosage:

Apply it to the affected part and change the dressing every 1—3 days

Oral Administration

Ingredients:

Helwingia japonica root, eucommia bark, *pterismultifida*

259

and root of *alangium chinensis* 9 grams each; giant knotweed, a-canthopanax bark, *chloranthus henryi* and root of *gynura bodie-nieri* 6 grams each; chuanxiong rhizome goldthread root, licorice root, safflower dried stem of *paris polyphylla* and rhizome dry-nariae 3 grams.

Pharmaceutical Process:

Let the above herbs infuse in 500 grams of spirits for 3—5 days

Indication:

Fracture

Administration and Dosage:

Oral administration, 10-20ml. doses, 2 or 3 times per day

Source:

Selection of Materials of National Exhibition of Chinese Herbal Medicine and New Therapy 1972, p. 313. (Yanshan Coun-ty, Wenshan Zhuang Autonomous Region of Yunnan Province)

2. *Sambucus* Spirit

Ingredients:

Fresh root of *sambucus williamsii*

Pharmaceutical Process:

Pound the herb and add proper amount of sweet wine or spirits.

Indication:

Fracture, dislocation of joints

Administration and Dosage:

Apply it to the affected part after reduction, changing the dressing every three days. The fracture will be healed after 1—3 times.

Source:

Selection of Materials of National Exhibition of Chinese Herbal Medicine and New Therapy 1972, p. 324. (Chaoyang Co-operative Clinic of Guiyang City, Guizhou Province)

3. *Sargentodoxa* Spirit

Ingredients:

Dried stem of *sargentodoxa cuneata* 2 kilograms, eucommia bark 2 kilograms, *cynura divaricata* root 1.5 kilograms, *zanthoxylum climorphophyllum* root 1.5 kilograms, *zanthoxylum planispinum* 1.5 kilograms, branch of *uncaria rhynchophylla* 1.5 kilograms, *alpinia japonica* 1.5 kilograms, leaves of *bauhinia championi* 1.5 kilograms, *ribes henryi* root 2.5 kilograms, Japanese polygala 0.5 kilogram, panax pseudo-gingseng root 50 grams, *cocculus trilobus* leaves 1 kilogram, *dysosma pleiantha* root 1 kilogram, *periploca calophylla* stem 1 kilogram, Dashuyao 2 kilograms

Pharmaceutical Process:

Let the herbs infuse in 60 kilograms of spirits

Indication:

Fracture

Administration and Dosage:

Oral administration for severe cases, 15 gram doses, 2 or 3 times per day

Caution:

Pregnant women must not take it

Source:

Selection of Materials of National Exhibition of Chinese Herbal Medicine and New Therapy 1972, p. 322 (Qiannan Hospital of Traditional Chinese Medicine, Guizhou Province).

4. Desmodium Spirit

Ingredients:

Desmodium

Pharmaceutical Process:

Ⅰ. Pound 1,000 grams of desmodium leaves into pulp, stir-bake it with a little alcohol till the color turns light yellow, then put it into water and decoct it over a slow fire for 6-8 hours. Wring out the juice and filtrate it, mix the filtrate with a certain amount of spirits to obtain 500ml of 43% proof spirits. Ⅱ. Wash and clean desmodium leaves and mince them. Submerge them in water, decoct them for two hours, then for half an hour. Mix the decoctions and concentrate the mixture to the proper amount, add 45% proof alcohol to make its alcohol content at 50-60% and the herb content at 1 : 1 or 1 : 2. Keep the mixture static for 24 hours and then filtrate it.

Actions:

Promotes reunion of bones, muscles and ligments.

Indication:

Fracture.

Administration and Dosage:

After manual reposition, apply the spirits to the fractured part and put on a small splint for external support (traction can be maintained if needed). Drip the spirit into the gauze under the splint every day. 50ml for adults, 30ml for children, once or twice per day.

Source:

Hainan Hygiene No. 4, 1976, p. 19, Haikou Hospital of

Hainan Farming, Hainan Province

5. Spirit of *Dipsaci* and *Pyritum*

Ingredients:

Dipsaci root 30 grams, calcined *pyritum* 60 grams, spirits 500 grams

Pharmaceutical Process:

Soak the herbs in the spirits for 7 days

Indication:

Fracture

Administration and Dosage:

Oral administration according to one's capacity for alcohol

Source:

Chinese Medicated Dietetics 1985, p. 227

6. Rooster Blood Spirit

Ingredient:

One rooster

Pharmaceutical Process:

Stab the roosten for blood, mix the blood with certain amount of spirits according to one's capacity

Indication:

Fracture

Administration and Dosage:

Immediate oral administration

Source:

A Handbook of Family Dietetic Therapy 1982. p. 202

Section Forty-seven Osteomyelitise

It is very difficult to cure osteomyelitise which is usually caused by deficiency of the kidney and bone, retention of phlegm and fluid or metastatic abscess. Traditional Chinese medicine categorizes it as phlegm of *yin*.

1. Rhododendron Spirit

Oral Admimistration

Ingredients:

Root of *rhododendron delavayi* 120 grams

Pharmaceutical Process:

Let the herb infuse in 500 grams of spirits for three days

Indication:

Chronic osteomyelitise

Administration and Dosage:

Oral administration, 15-20ml. in the morning and in the evening. Children can take a smaller dose.

External Treatment

Ingredients:

Colla Corii Asini

Pharmaceutical Process:

Put it into a proper amount of water and let it dissolve over a slow fire. Evaporate the water as much as possible and reel off threads according to the size of the fistula, then cool them on glass. When they are hard again, put them in sterilized gauze and get them ready for use

Administration and Dosage:

Wash and clean the affected part with potassium permanganate or hydrogen peroxide solution. Dip one end of the herb thread in boiling water to make it soft and fill the fistula with it, then wrap and fix the part with gauze. Change the dressing every

1-2 days.

Source:

Selection of Materials of National Exhibition of Chinese Herbal Medicine and New Therapy 1972, p. 326. (Yangguang Cooperative Clinic, Tonghai County, Yunnan Province)

2. Osteomyelitise Spirit

Ingredients:

Arnebia saxatilis and *lonicera confusa* 12 grams each; glorybower leaves 15 grams, *spatholobi* stem, *gastrodiaelata* root and sappan wood 9 grams each; *saururus chinesis*, whitefish and white rose of sharon 6 grams each; Bijiteng 12 grams, Wuyuehong 18 grams

Pharmaceutical Process:

Decoct the herbs together in 500 grams of spirits (or red wine); or decoct the herbs in water in case the patient cannot drink alcohol

Indications:

Subacute of chronic osteomyelitise, osteotuberculosis

Administration and Dosage:

Oral administration, half a dose each time and twice per day for adults; after five or six doses, decoct the remaining spirit with a pig's trotters and drink the decoction

Source:

Selection of Materials of National Exhibition of Chinese Herbal Medicine and New Therapy 1972, p. 326. (People's Hospital of Fuan Prefecture, Fujan Province)

3. Hemp Seed Spirit

Ingredients:

Hemp seed kernels

Pharmaceutical Process:

Parch the kernels till they smell good, then put them into a bag and let them infuse in spirits.

Indications:

Wind-toxic pain of bone marrow, even the pain of those who are unable to move

Administration and Dosage:

Oral administration according to one's capacity for alcohol

Source:

A Handbook of Family Dietetic Therapy 1982, p. 512

4. Frog Spirit

Ingredients:

One frog, brown sugar and spirits 100 grams each; stemonae root 15 grams

Pharmaceutical Process:

Decoct the above ingredients together

Indication:

Osteotuberculosis

Administration and Dosage:

Oral administration, one dose each time and once per day

Source:

Materials of New Therapy with Chinese Herbal Medicine, (Inner Monqolia)

Section Forty-eight Cancer

Cancer is malignant tumor which may occur in any part of the body. It has various clinical symptoms.

1. Airpotato Yam Spirit

Ingredients:

Airpotato yam 300 grams, proper amount of spirits

Pharmaceutical Process:

Pulverize the herb and put it into a container, add solution of prescribed amount and cover the container. Let the herb infuse for several days, then pour out the clear infusion of the upper part, and put more solution into the container. Let the herb infuse till it does not have any medicinal smell and get more infusion in the same way. Mix the infusions, keep them static for two days, then filtrate the mixture. Add more spirits through the filter till it amounts to 1000ml

Actions:

Removes toxic substance and heat from the blood, subdues swelling and removes masses

Indication:

Esophagas cancer

Source:

News Reports on New Medicine Issue 2, 1972, p. 24).

2. Chinese Actinidia Spirit

Ingredients:

Chinese actinidia root 250 grams, proper amount of spirits

Pharmaceutical Process:

Infuse the herb in the spirits for 7 days

Indication:

Digestive tract cancer

Administration and Dosage:

15-30ml. three times per day, oral administration

Source:

A *Handbook of Family Dietetic Therapy* 1982, p. 93

3. Pumpkin Spirit

Ingredients:

Two fruit bases of pumpkins, 100 grams of yellow rice wine

Pharmaceutical Process:

Burn the bases with their original properties retained, grind them into fine powder and take it with yellow rice wine

Indication:

Mastocarcinoma

Administration and Dosage:

Oral administration, twice per day in the morning and in the evening

Source:

A *Handbook of Family Dietetic Therapy* 1982, p. 59

4. Wine of Toad

Ingredients:

30 grams of live toad and 500 grams of yellow rice wine

Pharmaceutical Process:

Decoct the toad in the rice wine for 30 minutes, remove the toad and keep the wine in a cool place

Indication:

Liver cancer

Administration and Dosage:

Oral administration, 10 ml doses, three times per day for thirty days; after three days' pause, continue for another three months, which constitutes one course of treatment

Source:

Section Forty-nine Goitre Tumor and Scrofula

The clinical symptoms of goitre tumor are obvious thickening of the neck which feels heavy, tight and strained. In modern medical science, it is called simple goitre and is due to lack of iodine.

Scrofula usually occurs at both sides of the neck or behind the ears or below the cheeks. It is so called since tubercules hang around like chains of pearls. In modern medicine, it is called lymphatic tuberculosis and lymphosarcoma, etc.

1. Spirit of Marine Algae

Ingredients:

Marine algae 500 grams, spirits 1000ml

Pharmaceutical Process:

Put the algae into a silk bag and let it infuse in the clear spirit for 2 days in spring or summer, or three days in autumn or in winter. When the spirits dry up , dry and grind the dregs into fine powder.

Indications:

Scrofula and goitre

Administration and Dosage:

20ml doses, three times per day

Source:

A Handbook of Family Dietetic Therapy (1982, p. 84).

Section Fifty   Frostbite

Frostbite is a skin disease caused by longtime exposure to cold. It causes local purplish erythema or hard lumps or even swelling and blisters in severe cases.

1. Pepper Spirit

Ingredients:

Peppercorn 10%, spirits 90%

Pharmaceutical Process:

Let the corn infuse in the spirit for 7 days and filtrate the infusion.

Indication:

Frostbite

Source:

Selection of New Therapy with Chinese Herbal Medicine (Neimenggu)

Section Fifty-one   Anesthesia

1. *Murraya Paniculata* Spirit

Ingredients:

500 grams of fresh leaves and branches of *murraya paniculata*

Pharmaceutical Process:

Wash the leaves clean, pound them into pulp, then let it infuse in Sanhua spirit of 1000ml for 24 hours and filtrate the infusion

Action:

Anesthesia

Indication:

Tonsillectomy

Administration and Dosage:

Apply it directly to the mucous membrane of the throat,

Anesthesia occurs several minutes later and lasts for about ten minutes.

Source:

National Collection of Chinese Herbal Medicines Vol. 1, 1973, p. 19. (People's Hospital of Guangxi Zhuang Autonomous Region)

Section Fifty-two   Ophthalmic Diseases

1. *Curcumae* Spirit

Ingredients:

Scutellaria root, rhuburb, capejasmine fruit, Chinese angelica root, *curcumae* root, chuanxiong rhizome, red peony root, ledebouriella root, gentiana root

Pharmaceutical Process:

Grind all the herbs into fine powder and mix it with spirits for oral administration

Indications:

Aching eyeball, greenish-white pupil, sudden protrusion of pupil

Administration and Dosage:

Take 9 grams with spirits each time after meals twice per day

Source:

Collection of Fine Prescriptions

2. Wolfberry Spirit

Ingredients:

200 grams of Chinese wolfberry fruit and 600ml spirits

Pharmaceutical Process:

Cut the washed fruit into pieces, then put them into a bottle together with 400ml of the spirit, seal the bottle and let them infuse for one week, shaking the bottle once a day.

Actions:

Nourishes the liver and kidneys.

Indications:

Dryness and discomfort of the eyes, blurred vision, amblyopia, lacrimation against wind, muscular atrophy, pale complexion

Administration and Dosage:

Oral administration, 10-20ml once per day before supper or sleep. Replenish the bottle with the remaining 200ml spirits as the spirit in the bottle is reduced and mix the infused wolfberry fruit with sugar for oral administration.

Source:

Peaceful Holy Benevolent Prescriptions

3. Chrysanthemum Wine

Ingredients:

Chinese wolfberry root, dried rehmannia root 1,000 and chrysanthemum flower 1,000 grams each.

Pharmaceutical Process:

Decoct the above herbs together in water and use the decoction to make wine with polished glutinous rice and distiller's yeast

Actions:

Nourishes the liver and improves eyesight

Indication:

Blurred vision

Administration and Dosage:

272

30ml doses, twice per day

Source:

Peaceful Holy Benevolent Prescriptions

Section Fifty-three　　Infantile Paralysis

Infantile paralysis, also called poliomyelitis in modern medicine, is an acute infectious disease, Its clinical symptoms include: pyrexia, pains in the limbs, together with symptoms in the respiratory and gastrointestinal tracts, even acroparalysis and flaccid paralysis. This disease is mostly seen among children of 1-5 years old.

1. Centipedae Spirit

Ingredients:

60 grams of centipedae

Pharmaceutical Process:

Let the herb infuse in a sealed container for two hours

Indication:

Infantile paralysis

Administration and Dosage:

Apply it to the affected part and rub the part for 15-30 minutes each time, 3-5 times per day

Source:

Selection of Materials of National Exhibition of Chinese Herbal Medicine and New Therapy (1972, p. 37, Hospital of Chennan Commune of Li County, Hunan Province)

Section Fifty-four　　Toothache

Toothache is a common disease and can be caused by many

factors.

1. Spirit of Aconite and *Clematis Lasiandra*

Ingredients:

Raw wild aconite root 9 grams; *achillea alpina* and borneol 6 grams each; *clematis lasiandra* 30 grams

Pharmaceutical Process:

Grind the above herbs into fine powder and infuse it in 500 grams of spirits for one week

Indications:

Toothache, ache due to pulpitis, peridentitis, pericementitis

Administration and Dosage:

Dip the absorbent cotton in the spirits and apply it to or tuck it into the painful part once per day

Source:

Selection of Materials of National Exhibition of Chinese Herbal Medicine and New Therapy 1972, p. 396. (Wenahan, Yunnan Province)

Section Fifty-five   Osteoarthrosis Deformans Endemica

It is a regional disease and usually found in the northwest and northeast parts of China. Main symptoms are pain in the limb joints, enlarged and twisted joints, muscle atrophy, and consequent hampering of movement.

1. Pine Branch Spirit

Ingredients:

Nodular branch of pine 7.5 kilograms, mushroom 750 grams, safflower 500 grams

Pharmaceutical Process:

Decoct the above herbs in 50 kilograms of water and boil them dowm to 25 kilograms, filtrate the decoction and remove the dregs, then add 50 kilograms of spirits to the filtrate

Indication:

Osteoarthrosis, deformans endemica

Administration and Dosage:

20ml doses, twice per day orally.

Source:

Selection of Materials of National Exhibition of Chinese Herbal Medicine and New Therapy 1972, p. 194. (Qinyuan County, Shanxi Province)

Section Fifty-six   Leprosy

Leprosy is a chronic infectious disease caused by lepromin.

1. Multiflower Knotweed Spirit

Ingredients:

Multiflower knotweed root 120 grams, Chinese angelicae root, Chinese angelica root-tip, dried rehmannia root, prepared rehmannia root and *ranalimnocharis Boie* 30 grams each; aconite root (macerated and peeled), wild aconite root (macerated and peeled), acanthopanax bark, dried pine needles and biotae tops 12 grams each; prepared pangolin scale 30 kilograms.

Pharmaceutical Process:

Put the above herbs into a cotton bag, tie up the mouth, put the bag together with 10 kilograms of yellow rice wine into a jar, decoct them in water for two or three hours and keep them underground for 7 days.

Indication:

Leprosy

Administration and Dosage:

Oral administration. Take a dose enough to get drunk each time and keep away from wind.

Source:

Medical Treasure Collection. Gist of Surgwry (73rd prescription)

Section Fifty-seven   Spirit to Dispel Epidemic Pathogenic Factors

"Yili,"a term of traditional Chinese medicine, refers to those noxious atmospheric influences which are infectious and epidemic and are strong enough to cause diseases and great harm.

1. *Tusu* Spirit

Ingredients:

14 red beans, platycodon root, rhuburb, smilax China root and *pericarpium zanthoxyli* 15 grams each; ledebouriella root 30 grams, cinnamom bark 22. 5 grams, aconite root 7. 5 grams

Pharmaceutical Process:

Put the above herbs into a purple triangular bag and hang it in the lower part of a well on New Year's Eve. Take it out on New Year's Day and infuse it in spirits, and bring the herbs to the boil several times.

Actions:

Dispels and prevents epidemic pathogenic factors

Administration and Dosage:

Oral administration according to one's capacity for alcohol

Source:

A Handbook of Family Dietetic Therapy 1982, p. 510 (Chen Yanzhi said: It is a recipe by Huatuo. One can be prevented from all impure pathogenic factors by drinking medicinal spirits prescribed by it on New Year's Day.)

Section Fifty-eight　　Getting Rid of Fishbones

People may get fishbones stuck in their throats if they are not careful enough when eating fish. One should go to a doctor to have it removed surgically if the case is severe. For a slight case, it can be treated in the following way.

1. Spirit of Clematis and Sugar

Ingredients:

Clematis root and brown sugar 30 grams each; 15ml of spirits.

Pharmaceutical Process:

Put the above herbs and the spirits together into a pot, add 400ml of water, then boil them down to 200ml and filtrate the decoction

Indication:

Fishbones stuck in throat

Administration and Dosage:

Oral administration, 200ml each time and once or twice per day

Source:

1,100 *Folk Prescriptions of Dietetic Therapy* 1982, p. 288

中国药酒

吕　磊　于扬波　编著
吕树芸　刘红军

李杨　姜晓梅　译

哈罗德·师文德　校译

*

中国山东友谊出版社出版

（中国山东济南胜利大街 39 号）

中国山东新华印刷厂德州厂印刷

中国国际图书贸易总公司发行

（中国北京车公庄西路 35 号）

北京邮政信箱第 399 号　邮政编码 100044

英文版

1996 年 7 月第 1 版　1996 年 7 月第 1 次印刷

ISBN7—80551—835—1/R·16

06800

14—E—3076P